One Student Nurse To Another
All In One Study Guide

Carol Gibb

carol@onestudentnursetoanother.com

Ordering Information:
Quantity sales. Special discounts are available on quantity purchases by corporations, associations, and others. For details, contact the publisher at the address above.
Printed in the United States of America.

DEDICATION

To all Nursing Students Young and Old

CONTENTS

ACKNOWLEDGMENTS

Thank you to all who supported me through the years. My Loving Husband Micheal and Best friend David who believed in me. To my son Kyle who encourages me to live life to the fullest.

Chapter 1

INTEGUMENTARTY SYSTEM

Introduction of the Integumentary System

Integumentary: organ derived from skin (hair, nails, and glands)
Structure: epidermis and dermis (corium), skin hypodermis known as subcutaneous or superficial connective tissue.

Function: to protect from dehydration, elements and to maintain normal body activities.

Epidermis: derived from Ectoderm keratinized stratified squamous epithelium 0.07 to 1.4 mm and consists of:
Stratum basale or germinativum
Stratum spinosum
Stratum granulosum
Stratum lucidum
Stratum corneum

Glands: derived from skin, sebaceous and sweat glands.

Sebaceous-simple branched alveolar (acinar glands with holocrine mode of secretion.
Sweat fluids contain ammonia, urea, uric acid and sodium chloride (eccrine and apocrine).

Eccrine-simple coiled tubular with merocrine mode secretion.
Apocrine glands are-large with merocrine mode of secretion.

Hair: filamentous keratinized derived from skin which consists of the hair shaft and root.

Follicles: have two sheaths-epithelial root sheath and connective tissue root sheath.

Growth of hair-depends on cells of matrix adjacent to dermal papilla in the hair bulb. The matrix cells binding the dermal papilla proliferate and give raise to cells which move upward, and become part of specific layers to the hair root and inner epithelial root sheath.

Musculature-associated with arrector pili muscles these muscle bundles extend from the dermal. Root sheath to the dermal papilla. Contraction results in standing up of the hairs.

Nails- keratinized epithelial cells on dorsal of distal phalanges of fingers and toes.

Dermatology:
Epidermis- dead slough skin
Dermis- TB and Allergy Shots
Subcutaneous- no need to aspirate. No nerves here.
Hair, Nails, and Glands

Functions:
Protection
Sensory, Tactile, Feeling
H2o Balance can excrete through skin and kidneys.
Temperature Regulation

Disorders:
Inflammation
Neoplasm, New Growth
Metabolic
Nutritional
Physical
Chemical
Microbiological, Diseases

Prevention:
Cleanliness-Note: no irritant soaps, through drying, Pathogens can enter easily.
Diet-Note: shallow color could mean malnutrition.
Age-Note: elders oil secretion is altered, two showers a week unless necessary and a clean environment.

Diagnostic Tests
Biopsy: for abnormalities
Inspection: assessing the skin
Diascopy: apply pressure with a finger or slide.
Culture and Sensitivity: Culture is to identify germs, Sensitivity is to find the best medicine for treatment.
Patch Test: scratch test for allergies.H1 Histamines, H2 Parietal.

Nursing Processing Assessment:
Check: Skin color and temperature, Integrity and or Edema.
Itching and or Pain
Take History for: rashes, allergies, lesions, soaps, been swimming or in the woods. Where it starts, what makes it better or worse? Description of the infected area. Document what you see, also where on the body it is. Inspect under arms and pubic area.

Nursing Diagnoses:
Types of Lesions:
Macule: Flat, Vesicle: Fluid Filled, Wheal: Raised, Plague: Dry Patch.
Impaired Skin Integrity
Pain
Risk for Infection
Self Esteem
Social Isolation
Sleep Pattern Disturbances

Assessment of Skin and Diseases

Assessing Skin Color and Possible Problems:
Mucous membranes and conjunctiva should be Pink.
Dark skinned clients check oral mucous membranes.

Bronzing or Tanning: Possible Addison's disease, Adrenal's.

Tan: Chloasma, mask of pregnancy shown on face.

Lupus: butterfly rash on face.

Scleroderma localized: thickening of skin

Yellowing Tan: Tinea Vesicular, fawn colored skin or yellow patches.

Yellow: Uremia, liver disease, cirrhosis, cancer, gallbladder disease, obstructive jaundice.

Dusky Blue: Arsenic poisoning, paler spots on trunk and extremities Central cyanosis with hypoxia.

Peripheral Cyanosis: Vasoconstriction caused from cold exposure or vascular disease.

Pallor: Anemia, also in conjunctiva and mucous membranes.

Vitiligo: Patchy skin Albino is generalized.

Red Polycythemia erythema dilated superficial capillaries such as rosacea.

Skin Diseases

Herpes Simplex-Type1 HSV: Viral Infection. Also known as cold sore or fever blisters, and can be transferred from oral sex.
S&S: Lesions on lips and or nares, tingling, itching or burning sensation can be the first sign of presence. Vesicles then crusts over. Teach that reoccurrences lie dormant in body and contagious without eruption.
Nurse: Contact Isolation

Herpes Zoster Type2: Viral Shingles
S&S: usually around torso back and or front most times.
Nurse: emotional support, and to prevent secondary infections.

Impetigo: Bacterial Infection
Staphylococcus or Streptococcal bacteria. Highly contagious.
Positive skin culture for diagnoses.
Observe for red vesicles and pustules, especially on face and neck.
Macules to vesicles, ruptures then crusts over.

Nurse: Contact Isolation, Strict Handwashing. Teach to sterilize linens. Provide meticulous skin care instructions; give support to child and family.

Ring Worm: Fungal Infection
Tinea Capitus: Ringworm of the scalp.
Patches of alopecia May take 8 to 12 weeks to clear.
Tinea Corporis: Ringworm of the skin. Oval scaly inflamed ring with clear center. Pets can carry this.
Tinea Pedis: Athlete's Foot. Avoid public showers; wear flip flops and cotton socks.
Tinea Cruris: Jock Itch.

Thrush: S&S; Itchy skin, breakdown and peeling.
Nurse: teach mom to sterilize bottles and nipples, proper medication applications.

Scabies: Parasite Infection Itch Mite.
S&S: Usually first seen between fingers and axilla. Scabies can occur anywhere on the body. With severe Itching, eggs are laid under the skin then spreads. Moist body parts and spread by close person contact. Isolated mite dies within a day or two.

Nurse: contact isolation, Personal hygiene, meticulous laundry habits.

Pediculosis: Lice parasite seen on scalp and hairy areas of the body.
S&S: Intense Itching,
Nurse: first check around ears and base of scalp. Mature lice are seen on scalp and hairline. Hatch every 7 days. Reoccurs without treatment and can spread to whole family and friends. Teach: to wash all bed linens hats and do not share combs.
Pubic Louse: human to human, shave off hair for best results.

Acne Vulgaris: Inflammation of the sebaceous glands and hair follicles of the skin.
S&S: Puberty increases sex hormones and stimulates sebaceous glands.
Nurse: Teach that sunshine, balanced diet, sleep, and hygiene helps.

Psoriasis: Breaks in skin that stimulates plaque.
S&S: plaque covered silvery scales on elbows, knees, base of spine. Psoriasis can also affect palms of hands and souls of feet.
Nurse: teach proper applications of medications, and sunlight.

Eczema: Infantile Inflammation of skin, atopic dermatitis. Not contagious.
S&S: Caused by allergic reaction to some allergen. Observe skin for redness, swelling, papules or vesicles. And rash accompanied by itching, oozing and crusting.

Nurse: Help identify the allergen:
Inhalant: dust or pollen
Direct contact: wool, soap or strong sunlight.
Injections: vaccines or insect bites.
Digestive: foods or formula's. Teach skin hygiene, keep dry, prevent baby from scratching, and suggest mittens.

Diaper Dermatitis:
S&S: rash from prolonged contact with urine and or feces, laundry soaps, frictions, and sometimes the change from breast to bottle feeding. Beefy red may be Candida Thrush Infection.

Common Skin Lesions:
Strawberry Nevus: Hemangioma erupts at 2 weeks old and usually gone by 2 years old.
Sometimes surgery is suggested but not recommended.

Port Wine Nevus: associated with Sturge Weber Syndrome, Neurological problems and possible seizers and or retardation.

Nevus Simplex: generally fade by two years of life, sometimes called stork bites, visual white heads on face.
Sucking Blisters are from sucking fingers in utero.

Hairy Nevus: dark brown and hairy which is usually malignant.

Infectious skin lesions:
Seborrhea dermatitis
Staph aureus infections
Scalded skin syndrome: caused from infection, peeling scalp and inside ears.

Assessing Burns Depth of Burn
Superficial Partial Thickness (1st degree)
Minor burns show damage to epidermis such as sunburn.
Bright red or pink, usually dry. No blisters, blanches to light touch but Painful, sensitive to air and temp changes.
Will heal on own in 3 -7 days. Keep clean, cool, and dry.

Superficial Partial Thickness

Moderate Partial Thickness (2nd degree)
Epidermis and upper layer of dermis damaged.
From slight contact with hot objects, liquids, steam.
Weeping, edematous blisters.
Usually heals in 12 to 14 days.
Keep clean, dry, do not break blisters.

Deep Partial with Blisters

Deep Partial Thickness (2nd degree)
Epidermis and deeper dermis damaged.
Waxy white (still elastic) or blistered, mottled.
Edematous, and painful.
Can easily convert to full thickness (infection).
Healing takes 3-4 wks, new granulation tissue up through hair follicles.

Full Thickness (3rd Degree)

Epidermis, entire dermis, and subcutaneous fat layer
Dry, hard, inelastic skin, shades of tan to black.
Painless, insensitive to touch (nerve endings destroyed).
Edematous, can cause compression of structures under the eschar.
Continued Eschar removal, dressing changes, and grafting is a long process.

Extremely Deep Full Thickness (4th Degree)

Tissue damaged down to muscle, tendon, and bone
Black and open wounds visible tendons, bones, Extensive healing time with surgical debridement, grafting, and possible amputation.

Burn Size

Extent determined by percent of total body surface area burned. Rule of nines is based on body surface area of adult. Use chart to draw in burns on admission. Patient's own palm is equal to 1% of TBSA= (total body surface area) .Use the chart specific for children – body proportions are different which are important to accurately assess burn size and depth quickly.

The Amount of fluid resuscitation and decision to triage to burn center will depend on the information from assessment.

Appearance

Major Burn patients will be transferred to burn center.

Partial thickness > 25 % TBSA-total body surface area.

Full thickness > 10 % TBSA-total body surface area.

Involvement of high risk area, and a preexisting disease.

Special Considerations of Burns

Head, neck, chest (pulmonary injury)

Facial burns: Heat can coagulate protein in corneas.

Consult an ophthalmologist.

Ears: skin thin, little protection for cartilage and will not grow back if burned or infected.

Neck, hands, arms, shoulders, feet, ankles, legs, hips.

Contractures can occur.

Perineum: high rate of infection.

Moderate Uncomplicated Burn

Partial thickness 15 – 25 %

Full thickness less than 10 %

Need to be hospitalized, higher risk, but no need to be in a burn unit.

Minor Burn

Adults: with < 15 % partial thickness burn in non-critical area

Or < 2 % full thickness is usually sent home.

Causes of Burns

Thermal agents 94 % - 22 % of these are from hot liquids.
A Main cause of injury in kids < 2 years old. Incidence are increasing.
Chemical 3 %, Electrical 3 %.
Also See Steven Johnson Syndrome.

Steven Johnson Syndrome

Allergic reaction to any medication, flu like symptoms – then rash, blisters, skin sloughs like full thickness burn.
Mucosa of GI tract, mouth, eyes can slough as well.

Age

Elderly have higher mortality with less severe burns because of less resistance to infection also less able to tolerate multi-system stress.
Also not able to escape, and have a longer exposure.
Past Medical History Burn patient is not usually alert to give history.

Burn Trauma

Causes great stress to other systems.
Cardiovascular, pulmonary or renal disease may increase mortality.
Check for drug use, alcohol use, and suicide attempt that could increase mortality.

Thermal Burns

Most common flames, steam, heat (hot surface, metals, and liquids), radiation (sunburn)
Most accidents in home are from carelessness! Alcohol use, senility, or psychiatric disorders,
Smoking, neurological disease put people at high risk, including Industrial and auto injuries.

Prevention

Nurses educate public about prevention and safety.
Support and enforce laws that require labeled flammable contents, electrical warnings. Encourage/teach fire safety – turn down hot water heater. No painting/flammables near pilot lights.

Chemical Burns

Damage depends on:
Concentration of chemical
Mode of skin contact
Depth of penetration
Mechanism of action
Chemical Burn Treatment

Pathophysiology of Chemical Burns

Varies depending on chemical:
Industrial-strong acids, alkalis.
Household-exposure or ingestion of cleaning chemical, solvents, or paint removers. Some destroy tissues by coagulation necrosis, causing vascular thrombosis.
As skin is destroyed it becomes like a thermal injury.

Prevention

Safety, handling and information of chemicals.
Knowing the proper use, and what to do if exposed. (MSDS).
Such as Store in original container, out of reach of children.
Poison Control Center number must be posted.

Electrical Burns

Electrical sparks, arcs, current, or lightening pass through body.
Tissue is damaged from heat of electrical current, as it passes through body. Safety procedures: Teach never to touch down wires.

Electrical Injuries

Necrosis of GI tract
Cataracts damage from protein coagulation in the eye.
In Muscle necrosis the dead tissue releases myoglobin in proportion to damage. Myoglobin is 02 carrying protein of muscle.
Released in blood, can clog renal tubules, and cause renal failure.

Pathophysiology

Electrical current follows path of least resistance tissues high in water (conduct electricity).
Damage is in order of severity: blood, muscles, skin, tendons, fat, and bones. Most of injury is internal. Can see entrance and exit wounds.
Electrical current – causes fibrillation, cardiac arrest, and cardiac damage.

Lightening

Entry, exit sites, and branching burn pattern through skin.
Also causes, tympanic membrane perforation, cataracts, peripheral neuropathies.
Tissue Injury
Blood and nerves best heat conductors, bone the least conductive.
Less than 113 F (44 C). **Tissue** damage does not occur, unless prolonged. (More than 6 hrs) more than 122 F (51 C), time is brief.

Initial Wound Care

Never apply ice to burn tissue, can cause vasoconstriction and more damage. Never apply ointments, butter, oils that will hold in heat, difficult to wash off, bacteria.
Do not remove clothing adhered to burn, unless its burning, contains chemicals, can cause bleeding. Remove belts, jewelry if permitted.

First Aid Teaching

Thermal- move to fresh air.
Chemical- brush off dry chemicals, do not wet unless instructed.
Take container to ER. Do not induce vomiting unless instructed.
Electrical burns remove from source, only if it does not endanger others. Need Power Company to turn off source.
NPO- nothing by mouth-may vomit, aspirate
Psychological support to victim, and family

Respiratory Function

May have inhalation injury or altered respiratory function may be result of other system problems.

Hypovolemia – major problem in early burn victim is within (12 to 18 hrs).possible Tachypnea with shock. Overload – receiving massive amounts of fluid, can put patient in pulmonary edema.

Respiratory Injury

Inhalation injuries – 70 % mortality

3 types of injury:

Upper airway - exposure to hot air (see damage in 6 to 12 hrs).

Small airway/alveoli – exposure to toxic chemicals (see damage in 7 to 14 days).

Carbon Monoxide poisoning the symptoms is seen immediately.

Carbon Monoxide

You will see symptoms immediately.

Severity depends on % of Hgb saturated with CO.

< 15 % HA, 20- 30 % nausea, dizziness

> 40 % decreased LOC (loss of consciousness).

Cherry red color is not a reliable gauge, occurs with high levels of poisoning.

Extent of Injury

Does not always correlate with amount of skin injury. Can die of minor external burn if pulmonary injury is severe.

Causes pulmonary failure, inadequate perfusion of other organs.

High risk, suspect if burn occurred inside a building (enclosed area).

Exposed to more products of combustion (heat).

Symptoms of Inhalation Injury

Tachypnea, Crackles, wheezing, and or noisy respirations.

Burns to face: hoarseness, red swollen mouth or darkened mucosa, singed nasal hairs.

Carbonaceous sputum or blood tinged.

Use of accessory muscles is a great effort.

Kid's respiratory arrest without warning!

Pathophysiology

Airways: loss of cilia and epithelium, capillary leakage.
Tissue: edema, bacterial invasion.
Results in hypoventilation, atelectasis, pulmonary edema (non cardiac), bronchopneumonia (48 hrs) The Body in hypermetabolic state, with increased need for 02, removal of wastes, large fluid shifts.

Vascular Function

Initially marked vasoconstriction, then vasodilation.
Increased capillary permeability, fluid and electrolytes escape through damaged skin, or trapped under full thickness eschar and Causes major hypovolemia. Hct increased due to loss of plasma in relation to RBC, Hgb decreased due to RBC damage or trapping.
Vascular Permeability

Cardiovascular Status

Have to monitor effects of fluid replacement.
Vital signs. Avoid hypo and hypervolemia

Renal Function

Keep cardiac output adequate to perfuse kidneys. Acute Tubular necrosis can occur if they become ischemic. Glomerular Damage.

Gastrointestinal Function

Pathophysiology-edema, hyperemia of mucous membranes, increased histamine release.
Gastric dilation, paralytic ileus, increased gastric juice production, gastric vessel dilation.
Curling's ulcer-high risk, acute ulceration of stomach and duodenum. High mortality rate with perforation, GI Hemorrhage.

GI Treatment

Proton pump inhibitors, H 2 blockers, NG, antacids to keep gastric pH > 7. Monitor bowel sounds, early feeding to decrease gut atrophy. Also signs of bleeding.

Metabolism

Can cause more rapid tissue destruction than any other injury.
Fluid evaporation causes cooling, body has to work harder to
generate more heat.
Increased cell catabolism-lactic acid release (metabolic acidosis)
Protein stores used for new tissue, negative nitrogen balance, see
weight loss, muscle wasting. TPN/lipids. When GI tract is
functioning–Use protein shakes and supplements. Strict calorie
count, monitor albumin, 24 urines, ketones.

Neurological Function

Restlessness – hypoxia, hypovolemia
Seizures – hyponatremia, drug reactions, septic spread of microscopic
emboli to brain.
Prolonged positioning in one position – peripheral nerve
compression (from tissue edema), and permanent peripheral nerve
deficits. Need frequent orientation.

Intermediate Phase of Burn Care

Patient has survived initial resuscitation. This phase lasts for weeks to
months. Can die from sepsis (the most common cause), or
respiratory complications. The patient is dealing with extreme pain,
with dressing changes, grafting, splinting. Psychological – mourning
loss of body parts, function, and appearance.

Sepsis

Inspecting wounds each dressing change.
Odor and color of drainage can indicate organism involved. Culture
wound per instructions.
Monitor for: temp (> 101), hypothermia (< 98.6), hyperventilation,
tachypnea, agitation, anger, and hostility.
Septic shock –experience multi-system organ failure.
Gram Negative Infection, Gram Negative Septicemia Spread to
Normal Tissue.
Health Granulation Tissue Becomes Black with Systemic Infection.
Infected Face
Blue/Green Pseudomonas.

Wound Management

Debridement – healing/grafting cannot occur until the wound bed is free of all the dead/necrotic tissue.

Have to have clean, red granulation tissue.

Debridement process: removing dead tissue.

Granulation tissue is cleaned, and grafts laid and used for deep partial thickness, or full thickness.

Mechanical Debridement

Accomplished hydrotherapy and wet to dry dressing changes performed by special burn team.

Pulling off old dressing will help deride.

Patient is placed in tub suited for extent of burn, isotonic with added electrolytes (NaCl, KCL) Agitator helps loosen tissue.

Washed with antibacterial soap, wash cloths, men shaved.

Removal of Old Dressing

Tub with Agitator and Lift, Plinth Scale, Hip Tub

Dressing Changes

Patients are weighed on a plinth.

Take burn patient to warm, sterile dressing room for the removal of dead tissue using scissors, forceps (less than 20 minutes at a time)

Antimicrobial agents applied to soften eschar.

Dressings

Each body part is wrapped separately (fingers, ears, and toes) to keep from joining together.

Temporary Grafts

Homograft's skin harvested from donor cadavers. Cut into strips, preserved in bottles.

Cover large full thickness burns that can't be grafted yet (too large an area for autograft, or not clean enough)

They may stay on for days or weeks. Eventually slough.

Decrease pain, help prevent infection, prepare site for autograft.

Biosynthetic skin substitutes
Artificial skin, Biobrane (silicone, nylon, collagen peptides).As effective as homograft, cheaper, easier to obtain.

Integra – Used when autograft are not available or for reconstruction surgery. It has a dermal and epidermal component. Has dermis layer that is laid down first, which induces organized regeneration of new dermis by the body. The upper silicone epidermis remains intact as the dermal layer degrades. Weeks later, the silicon is removed and the wound can be covered with thin epidermal autograft.

Permanent Grafts
Autograft – split thickness of person's own skin removed with dermatome. Use thighs, back, abdomen, scalp for donor area.
Skin is slit to increase surface area. Cells grow to fill in holes.
Placed on clean granulation tissue (full thickness wound)
Need to keep immobilized for several days.

Grafted Skin
Will never look or perform like "normal"
Severe itching with healing
Use no lanolin or alcohol, which cause blisters) Grafts are very fragile – protect from scratching, injury, sun, burning. The site will be sensitive to hot and cold. Can't sweat, avoid overheating. Takes 6 months - year to mature and become less red.
Nurse: teach the Protection of Autograft Sites. Healed Graft Site.

Donor Sites
Now a partial thickness–burn.
Very painful, the burn is covered with FMG – fine mesh gauge scarlet red (antimicrobial), and Kerlix.
Treated like other burn tissue.
Scarlet red fine mesh gauge will dry and peel off as new skin grows beneath. The Site may be used over and over.
Burr holes in exposed skull for new granulation tissue growth.

Potential Donor Sites
Exposed Skull, No Granulation
Granulation Growing Out of Burr Holes Made in Skull
Granulation Tissue Filling In, Autograft on Granulation Tissue
Healed Donor Site

Cultured Epithelial Autograft
Skin biopsies taken from patient's non-burned area (3 cm x 1 cm)
Sent to lab, individual cells are cultivated to produce sheets of
epithelial cells. New skin is only epidermal layer which is Very thin,
friable. Tears and, shears easily. The site is a High risk for infection,
and contractures.

Complications
Contractures – burned joints high risk for new tissue becoming
fibrotic. Need daily, stretching, ROM. OT makes splints.
Splinting of hands, arms, feet in extension is to prevent contractures.
May lose function, and need surgery to release. Kids may need
repeated surgery for grafting, tissue release as they grow.

Burn Scar Hypertrophy (Keloid)
Keloids are an Over growth of scar tissue. Abnormal amounts of
collagen occurring in dermis and subcutaneous tissue.
Related to depth of burn, length of healing time, age, grafting, and
race – African Americans are more susceptible. Keloids can decrease
with sustained topical pressure, custom fit Jobst garments, until scar
matures about (12 month).

Burn Team: is a Specialized, educated burn/critical care nurses,
clinical nurse specialists. Burn/trauma surgeons and anesthesiologists.

Tumors and Characteristics:
Basil Cells: slow growing papule, crusted in center.
Squamous cell: irregular elevated, sun exposure and usually seen on
head. Malignant melanoma: most serious, color varies, irregular
border, aggressive growth. Vertical growth is more aggressive than
horizontal.

Key Words for Asepsis and Infection Control

Microorganisms-small entity

Infection control-policy and procedures: to minimize risk of nosocomial infection.

Asepsis-free of pathogenic microorganisms.

Medical asepsis-clean technique inhibits growth and spread.

Surgical asepsis- destroys all microorganisms and their spores.

Spore-formed by bacterium in the presence or absence of oxygen-aerobic/anaerobic.

Disinfection-chemical to apply to inanimate object.

Antiseptic-substance to reduce or inhibit the growth of microorganisms on humans.

Reservoir-natural habitat of microorganism that promotes growth and reproduction.

Carrier-person or animal harbors or spreads an organisms cause decease in others.

Vehicles- how organisms are carried about.

Contamination-soiled, touched, stained, and exposed to harmful agents.

Fomite- nonliving vehicle example: stethoscope.

Vector-arthropod

Host- an organism which another lives and nourishes on.

Nosocomial infection- acquired while in hosp.

Virulent-strength of the pathogen to produce decease.

Exogenous outside body.

Endogenous-inside the body.

Center for disease control prevention-CDC- set guidelines for blood, body fluids etc.

Standard precautions- set of rules prevent spread of infection.

Isolation precautions-guidelines for transmission of blood borne pathogens, all body fluids except sweat.

Double bag-

Place one contaminated bag inside another with proper label.

Sterilization- to destroy all microorganisms including spores.

Infection control- guidelines control spread of infection.

Impervious- unable to penetrate example: sharps.

Key points for Asepsis and Infection Control

An infection can develop as long as the 6 elements of infection chain are uninterrupted.

A microorganism's virulence depends on ability of body defense system.

Increase susceptibility in immune system are- age, poor nutrition, treatments, and conditions.

Signs of local infection and inflammation are similar-inflammatory response may occur without an infection.

Surgical asepsis requires more techniques than medical asepsis directed to eliminating microorganisms and spores.

All patients are potential infected with Infection/ HIV.

Nurse success to prevent infection to disease is a aseptic technique. Nurse does not take sphygmomanometer/blood pressure cuff into Isolation room to be used on another patient.

Lack of proper handwashing is the cause of many infections.

Isolation practices prevent personnel and patients from acquiring infections and prevent transmission to others.
Gowns, gloves, masks, eye protection are worn with blood, infectious material or splashes spray or where blood is generated.

A patient in isolation is subject to psychologic/emotional deprivation because o restricted environment.
Standard/ precautions isolation to prevent spread of organisms and all body fluids.

Non intact skin, and or mucous membranes.
Surgical asepsis practices followed if procedures are broken skin, invasive to body cavity normally free of Microorganisms.

Bruises:
0 to5 days: red to purple
5 to 7 days: green
7 to 10 days: yellow
10 to 14 days: brown and gone in 28 days

CHAPTER 2

SKELETAL MUSCULAR

Skeletal Muscular System
Review of the Muscular Skeletal System
Motion
Support
Protection
Skeletal Muscles
Movement
Joint Stability
Posture
Body Heat- produces blood flow and expending energy.

Diagnostic Tests
X-rays: fracture, misalignment, no signed permit.
CAT: muscle, tendon, NPO 3 hours if dye is used, signature of consent.
Bone Scan: inject radioactive isotope, to look for cold spots to determine blood flow, signature of consent.
MRI: magnetic field, strong guidelines, weight is important to fit into tube 300lbs limit.
Arthroscopy: scope for joints, Ingham Medical developed this, can also repair thru scope, decreases rehab time.
Arthrocentesis: withdraw fluid also can look around.
Biopsy: tissue mass removal for testing.
EMG: muscle transmits for nerve impulses, painful electric current. Sedation is not given so nerves will react, recorded on paper called oscilloscope.
Lab Tests: RA & ANA- rheumatoid arthritis, autoimmune/anti-nucleoid-antibody.
Nutritional Needs
High Calcium: dairy products - usually have vitamin D fortified.
High Protein: Meats-cheese
Vitamin D: proper utilization of Calcium-dietary-fish, organ meats, eggs-sun-natural form.

Muscular Skeletal Relaxants: muscle contracts if injured- relaxers relax muscle.

Nursing Assessment
History
Family- check for muscular skeletal problems, fractures.
Nutrition
Menopausal
ADL activities of daily living

Physical
Gait: important to document
Posture: can patient maintain posture sitting in chair.
Kyphosis/Hunchback, Lordosis/Sacral, Scoliosis/Lumbar
Deformities
ROM-range of motion all body parts.
Muscle mass- symmetry, proportion to the body,
Hypertrophy/Muscle; Atrophy/loosing muscle, Normal/soft supple.
Strength-lift against resistance, symmetry in handgrips, leg lifts in bed
without covers over legs.

Preventing Contractures and Loss of Tone
Contractures are muscles that are not anatomical positions.
Gradual Mobilization- find patients baseline so you can increase
activity gradual.
Assistive devices-crutches, walkers, canes.
Exercise-ROM range of motion 3-4 min four times a day, give meds
in advance if needed.

Positioning/Lifting and Turning
Assess patient needs
Positioning
Foot boards, High top tennis shoes, Bed cradles, Trochanter roll, No
external rotation of legs.
Lifting and Turning
Turning-Log roll especially for hip fractures.
Lifting-Overhead trapeze- patient can help if possible.
Draw sheet- count on 3 to peers

Enough help!!! Orthopedic patients if can't move head. Use 3 people, head/shoulders/head are supported.
Can make bed easier from top to bottom instead of side-by-side.
Exercise:
Passive- nurse does it.
Active- they can do it with assistance, praise and educate the patient.
Isometric- stationary exercises in chair.
CPM- continuous passive motion, nurse can set up with Doctors orders with Pain Management.

Slings/ Splints to immobilize affected joint.
Monitor circulation and sensation- and neurological assessment.
Assess for pressure points for numbness, tingle, parenthesis, pulse distal from injury for circulation, color, warmth.
Swelling takes 48 hours to peak

Body Image Disturbance
Self-care Deficit r/t- related to: ROM
Impaired Home Management
Altered Role Function

Stressors - Sprain/Strain/Dislocation
Sprain: Partial or complete tearing of ligament.
Strain: Pulling or tearing of muscle or tendon.
Dislocation: Displacement of bone- joints subluxation, **pulling** apart.

Treatment*RICE*
R-est Sprain/Strain- more painful than fracture, takes longer to heal.
I-ice-1st 48 hrs, inflammation process takes 48 hrs. Ice causes vasoconstriction.
C-ompression- ace wrap keeps fluid out.
E-lavation- 1st 48 hrs helps fluid go back to heart.
Fractures -Signs and Symptoms-Pain, Swelling, Deformity, Discoloration.
Greenstick- half is bent, Simple-fine line crack.
Compound-broken skin- thru the skin.
Comminuted-crushed bones usually do surgery.

Bone Healing
Initial break fluid, blood clot develops (hematoma) Edema & Blood.
Inflammation
Osteoblasts: breakdown of old bone.
Osteoclasts break down of new bone.
2) Procallus: cartilage and osteoid- protects the healing area and forms a bridge.
3) Callus: completed- sometimes left as a bump from the fracture.
Remodeling-osteoclasts- ossification
Removal and Reorganization- body eliminates excess bone around sight -by stress motion and weight bearing.

Fixation
External-Casts. Joint above and below, Immobilizer -allows early ambulation.
Internal- Pins, Screws, Plates for immobilizer.

Traction
Skeletal: 15-30 lbs - Pin care- high chance of osteomyelitis.
Skin: no more than 5-10 lbs of weight.
Bryant's-Pediatric traction
Buck's: Lower leg- ace wrap around like a sling with weights.
Russell's: ace wraps to support knee.
Head: for vertebra alignment.
Pelvic: for low back-Velcro goes around waist and weights added.
Doctor orders for weight, then x-ray to see if in right position, if nurse removes weights hold leg as weights are taken off, take weights off carefully, and hold the pulley to avoid rapid movements.
1) Ensure continuous traction,
2) Maintain counter traction
3) See that the pull of. Traction is removed sometimes to go down for x-rays. Must have help to remove traction. One holds the leg in proper alignment before slowly letting go the weight very slow, and then pillows are used for proper alignment. After returning same but reverse make sure all weights are done evenly and slowly. Make sure weights are hanging free.

Neuro assessment = color, temp, pulse, and pressure areas. Pulse on both sides should be the same.

Traction and counter alignment are opposite.

Pins are used screwed into bones instead of ace wrap or both for traction, pins are more complicated.

Pin care via protocol facility.

Complications of Fractures

Shock from too much blood loss.

S&S: increased heart rate, cool clammy skin, pale, anxiety

Infection: especially if. Open - Local pain, purulent drainage, chills and fever.

Osteomyelitis: bacterial - **SERIOUS** can take year to treat maybe longer. Gangrene: foul smell, watery drainage, redness, swelling.

Delayed healing-decrease calcium for bones and protein for muscles.

Fat Embolism: Fractured Femur - Tachypnea, petechiae -, rash on arms, neck, chest, or abdomen,

Looks like measles (Hip is most risky)

Compartment syndrome- in perimysium, blood flow stopped from pressure. Watch for (Severe pain not relieved)

(ORIF) Open reduction internal fixation, (ORIF) much better than traction and used more nowadays.

Neurovascular assessment, Early ambulation=Early release.

Casts

Plaster, Heavy, Bear more weight, Last longer – shiny when dry 24-72 hours.

Fiberglass, lighter weight, bears weight dries within 30 minutes.

Cast Care

Assess: (color, movement, sensation) – also check temp, numbness,

Cover rough edges. Monitor for skin breakdown, neuro checks for color, temperature, pulse and pressure points.

Bivalving- cut out an area where pressure is causing a problem.

Immobilizers used for simple fractures.

Hip Surgery

Causes: Trauma-Degenerative changes-Arthritis

Types- Screws- Ball and Socket

Interventions:

Neurovascular assessment-cap refill, movement and temperature, head of bed **no more than 35°**

Assess for DVT- post-op check for **Holman's** sign (rapid dorso flex) Positive Homans' pain will be unbearable.

Measure circumference mark and document so next nurse knows where to measure.

Abduction: to Prevent external rotation.

Hip flexion < 90 ° -forever - important remember this, no bending over. Do not cross legs which can cause hip to come out of socket, assess home for toilet height and furniture. Sometimes use adductive pillows to keep alignment. Toilets and chairs are more than a 90 so the home needs to be assessed for adaptation.

Abduction: external rotation: take away from spine.

Adduction: internal rotation: towards spine.

Joint Replacement

Cause: Chronic, uncontrolled pain, Obesity-stress on joints, Arthritis-rheumatoid, osteoarthritis.

Interventions

Pain Management-medication; communicate with therapist so pain level is tolerable before PT.

CPM- continuous passive motion- doctor writes this order.

Arthritis

Osteoarthritis: (noninflammatory degenerative joint disease)

Pain and loss of movement deteriorate articulate cartilage exposes bone then grows spurs.

Rheumatoid arthritis: inflammatory- loss of synovial tissue (synovial fluid is decreased friction), ankylosis (loss of mobility) Inflammatory Genetic tendency, Autoimmune- body destroys cartilage, Deformity and dysfunction.

Treatment: Exercise- even if painful Sometimes injections-into joint will last a few months, decreases pain and inflammation.

Surgery for joint replacement.

Gout
Hyper uremia - blood uric acid is elevated.
Cause: alcohol -Uric acid crystals settle in joints called Tophi.
S & S:
Uric acid, tight red, inflamed edematous joint, extreme pain in joint.
Treatment: avoid alcohol, low purine (Protein) diet stay away from (organ meats, fish, and poultry).

Osteoporosis
Cause: calcium &/or estrogen deficiency-postmenopausal, inactivity-after the age of 20 more bone breakdown than bone building. Some contributing factors, are Smoking, excessive alcohol.

S & S:
Kyphosis-Height loss-Frequent fractures.
Weight bearing exercise like walking.

Amputation-Surgical removal of all or part of limbs.
BKA-below knee
AKA-above knee
Causes: Trauma, Malignancy, Gangrene bacterial infection-peripheral vascular disease, Diabetes.

Stage1 nasty looking,
Stage 2 -systemic death.
Interventions: Assist patient with sense of loss, Phantom sensations. Encourage early ambulation and self-care-Focus on strength and Fit for Prosthesis.

Musculoskeletal Conditions
Bone Growth: Best indicator of biological age.
Fetus bone begin as connective tissue to Cartilage to Ossification (cartilage to bone)
Progression: rate may differ.
Long Bones: continues until epiphyseal fusion occurs.
Sprain = Ligament- Bone / Strain = Muscle

Types of Fractures
Simple: Broken-Spiral - Twisted break
Compound: Through skin - Oblique - Slanted
Greenstick: Broken/ Bent-Commuted - Crushed
Complete: Transverse - Across
Pain, pulse, sensation, color, capillary refill, movement-
Compartment syndrome, Volkmann's Ischemia,
Osteomyelitis/pin care
Plaster Cast takes 24-48 hours to dry- Use palms of hands to
position.
Spica cast wraps around waist then down leg.
Fracture involving epiphyseal affect growth - REVIEW   R.I.C.E.
(Rest, Ice Compression, and Elevate - Traction

Rheumatoid Arthritis-Inflammatory disease-Symptoms vary
Systemic
Polyarticular > 4 joints
Pauciarticular < 4
At risk for developing Iridocyclitis. Course is chronic with remissions
and exacerbations (makes effects greater). Worse in morning "gel"
phenomenon- how long it takes patient to get out of bed.
Treatment: Drug therapy and exercise-Nonsteroidal anti-
inflammatory.
Nurse: Education-Medication, warm baths, joint exercise and rest,
proper body alignment.

Legg-Calve-Perthes Disease (Coxa Plana) - Blood supply to the
epiphysis is disrupted- ball above epiphysis necrosis/then rebuilds.
It also affects the development of the head of the femur.
Distortion of the head of the femur leads to-Imperfect joint and
degenerative arthritis of the hip (adult life).
S&S-limping
Intermittent thigh pain -may refer to knee and limitation of motion.
Treatment - weight bearing with femur in an abducted (outward)
position - to hold femur head within the hip socket.
Traction - Braces – Cast

Muscular Dystrophy a **Progressive** degeneration of the muscles.
Duchenne Muscular Dystrophy - most common type.
Sex-linked inherited disorders manifested in boys- Mother are most likely are gene carriers.

S&S: Delayed motor development during infancy, Waddling gait-Slowness in running or climbing.
Enlarged rubbery muscles, Hypertrophied calf muscles, frequent falling, clumsiness, contractures of the ankles and hips. Gower maneuver-Gowers' Sign (Hip Girdle Weakness).
Treatment/Nursing Care-Treatment: mainly supportive.
Passive exercise, bracing, weight control- Surgery for joint contractures- Psychological to deal with.
Nurse: encourage normal activities as tolerated- Support to family & referrals.

Spinal Deformities: Three types
Kyphosis: hunchback-outward curvature of thoracic spine.
Scoliosis: lateral S shaped curvature of spine -most prevalent.
Lordosis: inward curvature of lower spine.
Scoliosis:-two types
Functional- poor posture
Structural- change in vertebrae

S&S: Uneven hemline, difficulty fitting clothes, uneven shoulder level, protruding hip.
Unequal arm to body space

Diagnosis & Treatment
Assess by view from the back and bending at waist.
One side of back appears higher than the other.
Definitive Diagnosis-spinal radiograph
Treatment-Correcting Curvature
Pre-operatively care
Assess neuro-muscular as base line-Color, Edema, Temperature of all extremities.

Milwaukee brace 25-45 degrees for moderate scoliosis, if more than 45 degrees surgery metal rod inserted /from ventral/front.

Osteomyelitis:
Infection of the bone -Occurs more frequently in boys than girls.
Staphylococcus Aureus 75%-80 % more than 5 yrs
Haemophilus Influenza less than 3 yrs
May proceed a local injury to the bone, needle hitting the bone can cause this.
S&S:-Pain, possible limp- lots of exudate. Decreased voluntary movement- Limited ROM-Refuse to stand or walk.

Osteogenesis Imperfecta:-Brittle bone disease-Inherited disorder of connective tissue.
Autosomal dominant, two types
Congenital: most severe, fractures and deformities occur in utero (Types II & III).
Tarda: frequent fractures of bones - frequently mistaken for Child Abuse (Types I & IV.) Some kids with type IV improve after puberty.
S&S:
Bone fractures: Bluish discoloration of the sclera
Osteoporosis: Short stature- Curvature of the spine
Abnormally short, bowed and deformed limbs
Elevated Serum Alkaline Phosphatase
Careful Positioning, Firm mattress
Genetic Counseling for affected families
Osteosarcoma- amputate is the choice
Ewing sarcoma

Review Axial Skeletal
Cranium:
Frontal
Partial
Temporal
Sphenoid
Ethmoid
Occipital

Facial:
Mandible
Maxilla
Zygomatic
Nasal
Lacrimal
Palatine
Inferior nasal conches
Vomer

Hyoid: hyoid bone

Ear ossicle malleus, incus, stapes

Vertebra
Cervical 7 C1 to C7
Thoracic 12 T1 to T12
Lumbar 5 L1 to L5
Sacrum 5 fused S1 to S5
Coccyx 4 fused

Thorax thoracic cage, boney thorax
Sternum1
True ribs 7 pair a side, vertebral sternum
False ribs 3 pair a side vertebrochondral
False ribs floaters 2 pair per side vertebral ribs

Appendicular Skeleton
Clavicle collarbone
Scapula shoulder blade
Humerus
Ulna
Radius

Carpals
Scaphoid
Trapezium
Capitate
Trapezoid
Lunate
Triquetrum
Pisiform
Hamate
Metacarpals
Phalanges
Pollex

Pelvic girdle hip
Coxal os coxae hip bones
Ilium
Ischium
Pubis

Lower Extremities
Femur
Patella
Tibia
Fibula

Tarsal
Talus
Calcaneus
Cuboid
Navicular
Medial cuneiform
Intermediate cuneiform
Lateral cuneiform
Metatarsals
Phalanges
Hallux

CHAPTER 3

DIGESTIVE SYSTEM

Gastrointestinal System and Accessory Organs

Accessory Salivary, Liver, Gallbladder, Pancreas
GI Tract/Alimentary: mouth, pharynx, esophagus, stomach, small intestine, large Intestine, anus.

Brief A & P

Accessory organs:

Liver gallbladder and pancreas. Mouth for mastication and teeth break down food. The Tongue pushes food back enzymes break down food goes from the esophagus to stomach.

Top of stomach is the cardiac sphincter or gastro esophageal sphincter. Prevents reflux, ph is acidic in stomach hydrochloric acid brakes things down. Stomach is a reservoir, hydrochloric acid factor gastrin and intrinsic factor solid to liquid Chyme. End of stomach is the pyloric sphincter that releases Chyme to the small intestine where ph is alkaline and enteric meds works here not in the stomach. Sustained release meds works in stomach and intestine.

Small intestine: duodenum, jejunum, ileum, bile and pancreatic enzymes which are amylase lipase and trypsin to break down to a more liquid state. Nutrients are absorbed in small intestine. End of small intestine is the ilio cecal valve.
Appendix has no known reason. Large intestine /colon major response of the large intestine is to retain water electrolytes and good bacteria. Rectum has internal and external sphincters Gastro colic reflux for defecation.

Liver, gallbladder (stores bile), pancreas- exocrine/amylase, lipase, traipse, endocrine/insulin, glucagon.

Diagnostic Studies: Ultrasound (Noninvasive), Cholangiography-visual gallbladder, CT (commuted Tomography).
ERCP- esophageal retrograde cholangiogram – NG tube to stomach to portal or ampulla of Vater to see stones.
Post op-check for gag reflex. A failing liver is unable to detox ammonia / breakdown of protein. Excessive Ammonia in blood causes Nero problems including Hepat Coma.

Nursing Process
History- family problems, meds, alcohol, diet, skin, itch, or yellow skin, does it bother you after eating.
Physical: skin, sclera of eyes, ascites (fluid in peritoneum) due to liver disease.

Nursing Diagnoses
Pain, Fluid Volume Deficit, Diarrhea, Bowel Incontinence, Alteration in Nutrition, Ineffective individual coping.

GI Accessory Organs/Stressors
Gallbladder: Cholelithiasis; Cholecystitis
Liver: Hepatitis; Cirrhosis
Pancreas: Pancreatitis; Cancer

Gallbladder: Cholelithiasis Possible Causes.
Multiple pregnancies and oral contraceptives, High cholesterol.
History: Extensive bowel resection or Crohn's disease
S & S- pain after eating, Indigestion, nausea after eating.
Jaundice, clay colored stools.
Treatment: Low-fat diet or possible Surgery.

Cholecystitis
Diagnosis: IV cholangiography- looking for inflammation or swelling.
S & S: severe pain in GB region (biliary colic) referring to sub scapula region. Vomiting- chills and fever.
Treatment: Lithotripsy, Surgery-Laparoscopic or Cholecystectomy.

Drains
Penrose: is not sutured, place 4x4 dressing to absorb fluid from drain. Dressing wicks fluid off, do not remove all the dressing when changing as may pull tube out. Clamp 1 hour before and after meals so bile can help digest food.
Sometimes patient is sent home with drain
Nurse: Assess -bowel sounds and stool.

Liver-Hepatitis
Causes-Viral
Preventative: immunization- Hep B only covers specific incident not a preventative to all.
S & S-Initial: flu like symptoms-Jaundice-Clay colored stool- Dark foamy urine.
Preventative: Passive Immunity-Immunoglobulin, hand washing, avoids sharing IV, tattoos.
Standard Precautions

Nursing Care-

Hepatitis A (viral)-MUST be reported-Supportive care.
Incubation Periods:
3-5 weeks **A** -Resolves itself. Infectious- from fecal route,
From not hand washing, possible contaminated water and food.
2-5 months **B**-infectious even 4-6 months after, Blood born, from sex, needle, lives along time 1-6 months.
7 Weeks Hepatitis **C**-Blood to Blood, from: tattoos, IV drug use 1-2 week onset, some can be carriers.
1-6 months Hepatitis **D**-Must have B - RNA virus through skin or mucous membranes.
3-6 weeks Hepatitis **E**-from fecal oral route water, food.

Cirrhosis: The liver can heal itself, once fat cells appear no chances of recovering. Liver biopsy checks for fat cells. Liver biopsy 6-7th rib supine position. Into liver inject NS to aspirate the cells for testing. Have patient lay on effected side. Post op. Monitor for lung puncture – all respiratory stressors.
Causes: alcohol 30-60 percent-Toxins-Viral-Biliary disease.
S & S-late in disease-liver palpable below R rib cage or elevated ALT and AST.
Jaundice-: ascites (fluid in abdomen) – neurological.
Manage ascites- restrict sodium -Na+ and fluid restriction; paracentesis-palliative process fluid returns.
Keep eye on labs as liver can't function and is able to develop toxicity.
Peritoneal Jugular shunt- tube inserted into belly and then to the superior vena cava.
Portal systemic encephalopathy-High levels of ammonia in blood.
S & S-delirium, convulsion, coma

Pancreatitis-Cause: alcohol; biliary disease.
S & S-severe abdominal pain radiating to back.
Diagnosis- shows an elevated Amylase.
Treat for pain management-Morphine Sulfate. Restrict fats-avoid ETOH. Pancreatic and Liver Cancer is usually fatal- usually 3 months to live.
S & S late in the disease.
Treatment: Transplantation- Liver-radiation and chemotherapy Pancreas debulk for palliative or Whipple's for comfort.

Gastrointestinal System and Stressors
Causes: Inflammation, Infection, Chemical, Physical, Structural, Genetics, Stress, Autoimmune.
Prevention: Nutrition- bulk maintains health of colon, drink water 8 glasses a day.
Nurse: Monitor and teach about Medication, Weight, and Cleanliness. Elimination- no straining, cause hemorrhoids or slow heart rate down.

Diagnostic Tests

Radiographic

UGI: swallow barium-NPO 8 hrs. POST op increase fluid, ambulate, stool white for 2days.

Barium Enema: can see colon, NPO 8 Hrs. laxative from doctor's orders the night before.

Endoscopic: visual esophageal, Duodenum NPO 8 hrs.

Colonoscopy: **visual colon**, NPO 8 hrs, post op assess for perforations, monitor for shock.

Gastric Analysis: test secretions and PH- NG tube, aspirate, and analyze content. **(5ml)**

High PH: gastric ulcers, low PH peptic ulcer, No PH cancer or pernicious edema.

Laboratory: Test- stool- occult blood test turns blue; red meat gives the test a false positive.

Nursing Process
Assessment:
History- trouble chew, swallow, flatus, nausea vomiting, indigestion, stools, appetite, diarrhea, bleeding, travel out of country.
Physical- skin discolor, abdomen for pulsations, 4quadrants in circular motion.

Nursing Diagnoses:
Fluid Volume Deficit
Alteration in Nutrition
Diarrhea, Constipation, or Bowel Incontinence.

Common Problems

Anorexia: loss of appetite
Causes: flu, meds, stress, taste buds and peristalsis decreased.
Physical or Psychological
Interventions: mouth care, rinse mouth, -variety of meals and
preference- eat slowly, small meals.
Nausea/Vomiting: Antiemetics
Assessment: Skin- turgor, Emesis-analyze, amount, appearance, how
many times and for how long.
Interventions: Ice Chips/NPO 6 hours-Introduce diet slowly/ flat,
Cool cloth-on forehead. Introduce clear liquids Small amount at a
time. If nausea and vomiting start again then go back to NPO for 6
hours and start over.

Flatus: use Antiflatulent
Assessment: what diet they are on.
Interventions: walking is best

Diarrhea

Increases peristalsis
Assessment: at risk patient -Characteristic of stool- how much, often,
color, consistency, odor.
Interventions: Limit intake food causes peristalsis-Privacy
Keep Area clean and dry add Vaseline to prevent abrasions.

Bleeding-

Cause: Varices- twisted veins, esophageal, alcoholics.
Blood backs up, pools in esophagus to the cardiac sphincter to
varices then bleeds.
Ulcers, Tumors, Polyps, Diverticula- Irritability

Assessment: vital signs check for Restlessness-Feeling faint.
Stool color- black sticky (melena) bright blood low bleed,
If blood is in stomach emesis looks like coffee grounds.
Is indication of a bleed is in lower stomach.

Laboratory

Hgb - Hct. Decreased Hgb and Hct, send soaked dressing to lab to determine if plasma loss or RBC loss.

Platelet count. Bleeding time, TCT= total clot time.

Interventions: Identify source

Upper-GI:

Enwall- is a Lavage for small bleeds.

Large bore tube, puts fluid in a bath/ aspirate, ice or room temp = vasoconstriction to stop bleeds.

Blakemore tube-NG tube, 3 balloons, inflate simultaneously, Deflates slowly to see if bleed has stopped, this is called portal hypertension. Lower GI- 1g drop in Hgb lost = 1U blood Transfusion, O2- saturation- Meds- antacids with small bleeds. Surgery. Hepatoencephalpathy- use reduce protein uptake, using, Lactulose is a cathartic (enema) and decreases uptake of ammonia from GI.

Dysphagia: difficult swallowing- Assess-types of food- suggest no dry food. Interventions: swallow evaluation, Sit upright when eating, chew food more, soft food, liquids with meals.

Eating Disorders

Anorexia Nervosa: underweight, electrolyte imbalance, stress, powerless. Want to correct electrolytes

Bulimia-binge/purge, usually dentist finds this as teeth are eroded.

Obesity

Stressors-Inflammatory
Appendicitis:

S & S-generalized not feeling well- Pain LRQ: lower left quadrant. Rebound tenderness: push down on abdomen and when released it pains, which is called – The McBurney's point.

Diagnosis: increases temperature, nausea and vomiting- Including. WBC increased bands = immature Segs.

Interventions-ice bag to site and surgery.

Peritonitis: Causes-ruptured appendix or ectopic pregnancy; perforated ulcers; trauma.
S & S: nausea and vomiting; Chills; Shock; Rigid abdomen.
Treatment-Broad-spectrum antibiotics are used.
Peritoneum is a sterile environment any time you get a leak in this area, and is irrigated with antibiotic solution.

Ulcerative Colitis
Diagnosis: presenting symptoms, endoscopy.
S & S: bloody mucoid diarrhea, pain-physical/emotional stress.
Treatment: nutritional, antidiarrheal s, analgesic, steroids, surgery.

Peptic Ulcer: Cause: low pH; H. pylori bacterium-genetics; stress, drugs, smoking.
Diagnosis: Barium Swallow; Endoscopy; Gastric Analysis, H. pylori.
S & S: epigastric pain, loss of appetite, spontaneous vomiting.
Treatment: antacids, sedatives, H2-receptor antagonist, Carafate Fills in ulcer.
Interventions: diet: restrict ETOH, caffeine, frequent regular meals.
Surgical Intervention: Pyloroplasty- repair pyloric, Vagotomy severs nerve decreases acid.

Gastric Resection
Subtotal- part of stomach
Total: all of stomach: esophagus anastomosed to duodenum.
Billroth I: distal portion of stomach removed anastomosed to-duodenum.
Billroth ll: distal part of stomach attached to Jejunum.

Cancer
S & S: weight loss, change in bowel habits, blood in stool (occult), abdominal pain.
Diagnosis: Stool, Barium Enema, Colonoscopy.
Treatment: chemotherapy (5-FU)

Surgical Interventions:
Hemicolectomy: to remove 1/2 of colon
Abdominoperineal Resection
Ostomies, Loop
Single-barrel: be sure bag is hanging with gravity at all times.
Double-barrel: depending on Location- possible reconnect.
Ileostomy: bypass whole colon, electrolyte imbalance is a big thing as no absorption of water, Fluid volume Deficit.

Intestinal Obstruction
Causes:
Mechanical: tumor, adhesions, twisting or telescopic, impaction-emergency surgery.
Symptoms: bowel sounds: high pitch, hyperactive to absent. Distension-pain corresponds to peristaltic wave, vomiting, and fecal smelling.
Interventions: decompress stomach, **Canter tube** (position changes), and weighted nasogastric tube for partial obstruction.

Hernia-Abdominal
Reducible: can push back in.
Incarcerated or Irreducible cannot push back in.
Strangulated: medical emergency as blood supply is cut off.

Hernia Hiatal-Pushes Through the wall of diaphragm and usually have signs of gerds.
S & S-belching, substernal pain, pressure after eating and increases lying down.
Diagnosis: UGI
Treatment-H-2 antagonist, proton pump inhibitor prevents reflux. Elevate head of bed, and do not eat before bed.

Diverticulosis/Diverticulitis-Diverticuli out pouch fills up with bacteria. Define: increased Infection increased Inflammation.
S & S: diarrhea, constipation, abdominal, Pain, fever, rectal bleeding.
Treatment: Teach avoid eating seeds, nuts popcorn, strawberries, tomatoes, celery, apple skin, alcohol.

Hemorrhoids

Define: dilated veins in rectum

S & S-localized pain and itching, bleeding

Treatment-Sitz bath, local anesthetic

Scleroplasty (inject normal saline to harden)

Cryotherapy

Photocoagulation

Rubber band ligation

Hemorrhoidectomy- must affect activities of daily living.

Gastrointestinal Conditions Child

Dehydration: Output Exceeds Input

Infants have greater % of water ECF (extracellular fluid) until age 2.

S & S: Infant weight is 1st priority for dehydration.

Increased Heart rate and Respiratory Rate

Blood pressure is normal or slightly lower.

Restless, irritable, lethargic or comatose.

Marked Thirst

Skin Turgor shows tenting

Skin, cool & clammy

Mucous membranes are extremely dry.

Anterior fontanel sunken

S & S Child

Increased Temperature

Rapid HR & RR

Skin cool & clammy

Mucous membranes are extremely dry.

Marked Thirst

Irritable, lethargic

Significance of Weight and Dehydration

Mild dehydration: 3% to 5% loss of body weight.
Moderate dehydration: 6% to 9% loss of body weight.
Severe dehydration: 10% or more loss of body weight.
Most important assessment is weight.

Vomiting is a Result of sudden contractions of the diaphragm and muscles of the stomach.
Persistent: dehydration & electrolyte imbalance.
Alkalosis: loss of hydrochloric acid
* Metabolic .7.45 and Increased $HCO3$.
"Spitting up" is a normal occurrence in infants & young children.
Projectile vomiting: forceful expulsion of the stomach's contents = obstruction.

Diarrhea

Infant – sudden increase in number of stools.
Change is consistency
Change in color – green
Blood or mucous
Infectious - Rotavirus, e-coli, salmonella or Shigella
Less than 2 weeks chronic malabsorption
Child – similar to adult
Watery stools, Explosive stools
Yellowish green in color
Treatment for diarrhea
Same for all age kids, Rest the intestine by reducing solid food intake.
Clear fluids: avoid broth (increased Na levels), Soft Diet (BRAT), Bananas, rice cereal, applesauce and toast with jelly.
Gradually return to regular diet (2-3 days)
Nursing Responsibilities: LPN monitors IV sight for patency and I&O
Interview parents/significant other about eating patterns, feeding techniques, frequency of episodes of vomiting or diarrhea, new foods added to diet.
Providing a non-threatening environment for the child,
(Stress of hospitalization increases the complications of dehydration)

Accidental Poisonings Review

Poisons commonly encountered in Pediatrics.

Tylenol: hepatic damage major concern. Induce vomiting or empty stomach.

Mucomyst (smells like rotten eggs) is antidote and given according to serum levels of, Acetaminophen is not given with charcoal.

Monitor VS, I&O and liver function test.

Omphalocele: Herniation through the umbilicus in which the abdominal contents and occasionally other organs protrude.

Sac is covered by translucent membrane may rupture at delivery.

Check for other anomalies.

Gastroschisis Herniation:

In the abdominal wall to the right of the umbilicus.

No membranous covering of the eviscerated contents.

Have few other congenital anomalies.

Esophageal Atresia/Tracheoesophageal Fistula (TEF)

Failure of GI tract to separate from the respiratory tract early prenatal.

Four types:

Isolate esophageal atresia: excessive salivation 8 percent

Esophageal atresia with distal TE fistula:

Excessive salivation, respiratory distress and reflux 86 percent

Esophageal atresia with both proximal and distal TE fistula:

Respiratory distress with feeding & reflux 1percent

Esophageal atresia with proximal TE fistula:

Respiratory distress especially with feedings 1percent

Diagnose by symptoms and confirmed by x-ray

Nurse – prevent pneumonia, choking & apnea

Esophageal Atresia 8percent

Esophageal Atresia with Proximal TE Fistula 1 %

Esophageal Atresia with Distal TE Fistula (86 %)

Esophageal Atresia with both Proximal &Distal TE Fistula 1percent

Isolated TE Fistula, H-Type 4 %

Imperforate anus Failure of GI tract & anal tissue to separate.
Meconium should pass w/24 hrs from birth.
Four Types
Type I: anal stenosis (5-6 percent) anus and lower rectum narrowed but patent.
Type II closed anal membrane (5-7 percent) anal opening covered by a membranous diaphragm.
Type III – Anal agenesis (85 %)
Type IIIA and Type IIIB
Type IV – anal atresia (3 percent) anal & rectal pouches separated by varying distances.

Celiac Disease: Gluten enteropathy/Sprue Inherited disposition with environmental triggers.
S & S present 6 months to 2 years when food containing gluten is introduced.
Failure to thrive. Large stools (bulky & frothy)
Diagnose: IgA serum
Treatment: Diet restrictions of wheat, barley, oats, & rye.

Hirschsprung's Disease Absence of ganglionic innervation to the muscle of a segment of the bowel.
More common in boys (1:5000 live births)
Problem occurs in the Lower portion of sigmoid colon.
Chronic constipation
Ribbon like stools, and abdominal distention.

Intussusception Slipping of one part of the intestine into another part just below it.
Can be life threatening.
Severe abdominal pain (loud cries)
Kicking and drawing legs to abdomen.
Vomiting (green-yellow), Bloody/mucous stools (after 12 hrs) looks like current jelly.
Rigid abdomen

Pyloric Stenosis
Narrowing of lower end of the stomach from an overgrowth of the circular muscles of the pylorus, and by spasm of the sphincter.
Appears 2 to 3 weeks of life, higher occurrence in boys,
and most common surgical condition of the GI tract.
Projectile vomiting – immediately after feeding contains mucus and ingested milk.
Dehydration
Surgical repair is suggested.

Thrush (Oral Candidiasis)
Infection of the mouth caused by fungus Candida.
Manifestations – white patches on gums tongue and roof of mouth cannot be wiped away.
Candid infection of the diaper area – bright red sharply demarcated diaper rash.

Worms
Pinworms (enterobiasis) most common in toddlers.
Looks like a white thread about 1/3 inch.
Pinworms come out of anus to lay eggs at night. Can spread rapidly from one person to another.
S/S: scratching the anal area & complain of itching.
Sample is taken at night from the rectal area.

Roundworms (ascariasis) * can obtain from the soil.
Asymptomatic or abdominal pain
May have chronic cough
Egg develops into larvae in the intestinal wall can go to the liver, lungs and the heart.
Asymptomatic until enter the glottis **cough up** worms swallow and start the cycle again.
Diagnoses: Eggs seen in stool
Treatment: Same as for Pinworm
Anti = against /Helminth = worms

Hernia

Inguinal Hernia: Protrusion of part of the abdominal content through the inguinal canal in the groin.

Umbilical Hernia: Protrusion of a portion of the intestine though the umbilical ring.
Will have surgery if bowel is compromised or may correct itself by2.

Diaphragmatic Hernia: Perfusion of the abdominal contents through an opening in the diaphragm
In utero –compromise lungs – intubate as soon as born.

Torsion in Testes-Axial rotation of the spermatic cord that cuts off the blood supply to the testes.
Epididymis & other structures (most common 1st yr & puberty)
Emergency surgery.

Gastrointestinal Assessment
Tube Feeding/Total Parenteral Nutrition.
GI Bleeding

Inspection: Color Lesions Scars Bulges Distension of superficial veins. Bruising on back (retroperitoneal bleed)

Auscultation:
Normal 5 – 35 sounds per minute
Hypoactive – below obstruction
Hyperactive – above obstruction
Loud gurgles – borborygmi
Rushing, high pitched – exaggerated peristalsis trying to push past obstruction. Listen in each quadrant for 1 min before determining bowel sounds are absent.

Palpation:

Light skin temp, masses, tenderness, guarding.

Nodes; location, size, consistency, mobility, tenderness

Deep: size and location of organs (kidneys, liver, spleen), masses

Aortic pulsations: (pulsing mass > 2 cm wide, directly above umbilicus)

Palpation: Don't palpate deeply, if there is pain with light palpation. Have person put their hand on yours to guide to where the pain is. They will feel in control and be more willing to let you palpate. Avoid where it hurts the most.

Fluid Wave

Test for presence of ascites.

Have someone place ulnar side of hand midline to dampen the wave,

Place palm on one side of abdomen.

And tap on other side and you will see fluid wave.

Nitrogen Balance

Neutral nitrogen balance - protein intake = output (NML diet and kidneys)

Positive nitrogen balance - intake exceeds output.

High protein oral, tube feedings.

Negative Nitrogen Balance

Nitrogen output exceeds protein intake.

Body stores (muscles) broken down and used for energy.

Inadequate protein intake (diet poor)

Protein not conserved - renal disease, protein leaks through glomeruli – proteinuria.

Increased need for protein.

Increased Need for Protein

Hypermetabolic states -burns, surgery.

Acute illness - fever, increased basic metabolic rate.

Long term illness - cancer, inflammatory bowel disease.

Immobility - need to rebuild muscles.

Tube Feeding Complications: Most common - nausea, vomiting, diarrhea. (H20 moves into bowel = hypertoxicity)
Problems - excessive volume, rate, gastric retention.
Hyperosmolar solution (especially when patient has Severe protein malnutrition albumin <3g/dL), (Normal 3.5 – 5. g/dl)
Solutions - Decrease bolus volume or rate dilute formula to isotonic; Gradually increase strength, warm, lactose free solution.

PEG Tube
Percutaneous endoscopic gastrostomy
The tube is placed via endoscope into the stomach.
Then a stab wound is made in the abdominal wall to pull the end of the tube through. A retention disk (or balloon) and external bumper secure the tube to the abdominal wall.

Total Parenteral Nutrition
Hyperalimentation
For patients who will not eat, or can't eat - abdominal trauma, surgery, possible bowel obstruction, sepsis, or coma.
Need to rest bowel - inflammation, pancreatitis • High metabolic demands (burns)

Composition
Peripheral - dextrose 5 – 10 %
Amino acids (protein) 2 - 3.5 %
Central - dextrose 15 – 50 %
Amino acids 3 – 5 %
Vitamins to metabolize glucose, protein, fat.
Electrolytes - Na+, K+, Cl-, Ca+, Phos
Regular insulin

Trace Elements
Copper, zinc – erythropoiesis
Iron – hematopoiesis
Copper, chromium - CHO metabolism
Zinc, chromium, selenium, molybdenum for enzymes.

Lipids

Fat - 10 - 20 percent solutions
Calories, essential fatty acids, can absorb fat soluble vitamins.
Reduces vein irritation from hyperosmolar TPN.
Only IVPB with TPN.

Complications of TPN

Fluid imbalances – hypervolemia
Monitor I & 0, daily weight, lung sounds, edema.
Electrolyte imbalances - K+, PO4+, Ca+
Pharmacy can add extra to each bag.

Sepsis

Solution high in glucose.
Central line breaks in skin, direct access to blood.
Patients may be immunologically compromised.
Monitor temp, catheter site, sterile dressing changes.
Port used only for TPN and lipids, increased. WBC, tachycardia, hypotension.
Metabolic
Hyperglycemia - High glucose concentrations.
This can cause hyperglycemic hyperosmolar nonketotic coma (HHNC) Check Blood sugar.
Check for High blood sugar, and dehydration.

Hyperglycemia

Treatment: Decrease glucose concentration, rate
Add regular insulin to TPN, sliding scale regular insulin every 6 hrs.
Increase lipid rate (more calories from fat, less from dextrose).

Lipid Imbalances

Hypertriglyceridemia - Transient after infusion of fat.
Lipids use egg phospholipids - do not use if allergic to eggs.
Monitor for rash, fever, chills (1st 30 min).
Rare: Dyspnea, nausea, chest or back pain, sleepiness, flushing, local irritation.

Fat Emulsion
Delayed reaction to lipids:
Hepatomegaly, thrombocytopenia, jaundice.
Fat overload syndrome
Leukocytosis, fever, splenomegaly, shock

Peritonitis
Inflammatory
Suppurative (pus)
Response of peritoneal lining to direct irritation or contamination.

Etiology
Cause can be GI or GU in origin
Perforations - peptic ulcer, bowel
Ruptures - gall bladder, appendix
Inflammation - Cholecystitis, pancreatitis, diverticulitis, leaking anastomosis.
Bowel obstruction could be a strangulated hernia.
Ruptured bladder
Reproductive infection

Pathophysiology
Chemicals - leaking bile, pancreatic enzymes, intestinal and gastric secretions, urine.
May be sterile at first, bacterial peritonitis begins within 6 - 12 hours.
Peritoneal lining - large semi-permeable membrane,
Injury/infection causes capillaries to dilate and leak.

Third Spacing
Hypovolemic shock
Dehydration decreased U/O, tachycardia, hypotension.
In the peritoneal cavity one can lose liters of fluid.
Fluid within the cavity impairs the function of Phagocytosis.
Microorganisms (E. coli) present begin to proliferate,
That produces leukotoxin that decrease function of leukocytes.

Septic Shock
Local becomes generalized.
Fulminant peritonitis within 12 - 24 hours.
Septic Shock
Multiple organ failure.

Cause of Organisms
Generally gram - (few gram + in upper track due to acidity)
Aerobic - E. coli, Proteus
Anaerobic - Bacteroides, clostridia
Fecal contamination - extremely high bacterial load.

Diagnostic Tests
Radiology - chest (esophagus),
Abdominal- (abnormal gas patterns, free air below diaphragm),
MRI, CT, ultrasound.
Angiography - vessel bleed, or ischemia.

Clinical Findings
Abdominal Pain, Guarding, Rigid, boardlike abdominal
Cough test – 76 percent grimaced, flinched, and moved hands to
abdominal. Rebound tenderness - may have some false positive.

Types of Pain
Parietal-Generally intense, sharp and localized.
Visceral-Dull poorly localized (no pain receptors in visceral
peritoneum, pain referred through visceral SNS).
Referred - felt at remote location (abdominal pain in shoulder -
Kehr's sign)

Systemic Findings
Chills, fever, diaphoresis
Anorexia, N/V
Tachycardia, tachypnea
Dehydration, low U/O
Restlessness, disorientation
Shock

Nursing Management
Assess pain - type, location, intensity.
Cough test, position change, rebound tenderness, rigidity.
Vital signs and monitor for shock.

Nursing Management
Monitor labs and bowel sounds.

Antibiotic Therapy
Cipro – broad spectrum
Flagyl - bowel organisms
Clindamycin – anaerobic
Cephalosporins - broad spectrum

Aminoglycosides
Aminoglycosides - aerobic
Gentamycin, Tobramycin, Vancomycin
Nephro and ototoxic

Fluid Therapy
To correct hypovolemic and septic shock.
Weight every day and measure the abdominal girth every shift.

Other Care
Semi fowlers, Best for respiratory, gravity promotes descent of infectious facilitates drainage.
Rest/Skin care

Surgical Treatment
Resect/repair cause (ruptured organ, perforation)
Drain abscesses
Resection, anastomosis of bowel.
Contaminated wounds open, abdominal wall held together - retention sutures.

Peritoneal Lavage

Surgery - > 3 liters of warm saline used to irrigate contaminated peritoneum.

Catheter may be left in post-op for continuous irrigation - NS and antibiotic (CAPD instill and drain)

Soft drains: Penrose (cover with ostomy bag if draining large amount), JP's.

Any retained fluid can cause infection.

Complications
Abdominal disasters!

Walled off abscesses (surgically drain),

Deep wound infections (abdominal cavity left open for irrigations and packing)

Retention "sutures" hold wall together.

Breakdown of anastomosis

Organ walls erode - fistula formation

Septic shock

Gastroesophageal Reflux Disease

Syndrome with reflux of gastric contents into the lower esophagus.

7% of Americans experience daily symptoms.

GERD Risk Factors Hiatal hernia

Incompetent lower esophageal sphincter (LES), Contents go from higher pressure in stomach to, lower pressure in esophagus. Affected by caffeine, chocolate, and anticholinergics. Decreased esophageal clearance from decreased esophageal motility, and gastric emptying.

Complications

Refluxed acids cause esophageal irritation, inflammation(esophagitis). Gastric pepsin, duodenal trypsin and bile salts corrode the esophageal mucosa. Changes to esophageal cells can cause Barrett's esophagitis – precancerous cells.

Esophageal stricture

Bronchospasm, asthma

Aspiration pneumonia

GI Bleeding

Upper GI: hematemesis (bloody vomitus) Fresh, bright blood – arterial.

Coffee ground look, darker, mixed with gastric juices - venous, capillary.

Lower GI - rectal bleeding.

Hematochezia - bright red, undigested blood – rectum, and may be mixed with stool or diarrhea.

Melena -Black, tarry, foul-smelling (ammonia) blood mixed with diarrhea.

Usually bleed higher up or slower bleed blood in system longer.

Occult - Blood not visible, detect with reagent.

No objective sign of bleeding – Patient. Presents symptoms of hypovolemia (syncope)

Diagnostic Procedures

Endoscopy (esophagogastroduodenoscopy, Proctosigmoidoscopy) This can visualize the lesion. May be able to use electrocautery or laser coagulation on bleeding vessels.

Angiography - Contrast dye injected to locate the bleeding vessel, And able to inject Keratolytic drug to scar vessel.

Chapter 4
Urinary System

Urinary System
A & P-kidney, bladder, ureter, urethra
Aorta to kidney to capillaries to Bowman's capsule to glomerulus to inferior vena cava.
Common Stressors:
Infections- UTI, bacterial
Diabetes Mellitus- arthrosclerosis which constrict BV's.
Circulatory Disorders, Heart Failure.
Obstructions, stones, masses, Hypoxia.

Prevention
Increase water
Hygiene-wipe front to back.
Control blood pressure- Keep in check more than 140/90 is bad.
Treat infections- cranberry juice and water will not cure infections.
Monitor Nephrotoxic drugs aminoglycosides, peaks and troughs.

Diagnostic Tests
Lab-BUN- blood, urea, and nitrogen increased dehydration or kidney disfunction.
Creatinine- number 1 test for kidney problems will show an increase.
UA, Culture
Osmolality- how concentrated the urine is.
Biopsy- cells

Radiologic Studies
KUB- kidney, ureter, bladder
IVP-pyelogram- looks at blood flow
Cystoscopy- view urethra and bladder
Renal Angiography- injects dye into the femoral artery looking for obstruction.

Nursing Process
History- of hypotension, diabetes, kidney stones, cardio problems UTI, problem empty bladder, frequency, nocturia.
Physical- check bladder for distension, palpate gently above pubic bone, color, clarity, odors.

Nursing Diagnosis
Fluid volume excess/deficit
Altered pattern of urinary elimination.
Pain
Sleep pattern disturbance
Body Image Disturbance
Knowledge Deficit

Common Problems- Incontinence
Types: Stress (laugh, /sneeze), urge (not in time), overflow (delay)
-neurological
Treatment- Bladder retraining.
Muscle exercises (Kegel)-tighten count 1-2-3 x 15 times 3-4x a day.
Catheter or Surgery

Nursing Interventions
Assessment of type and contributing factors.
Space fluids- no fluids few hours before bedtime.
Initiate bladder training- like baby x2 hours.
Patient Education- Kegel exercise strengthens the pelvic floor.

Common Therapies- Surgery called Cystoscopy
Catheterization
Straight- get sterile urine specimen if Unable to void
Unable to empty bladder
Clean catch-start stream then get catch sample (midstream)

Dialysis-Principle- Diffusion
Types
Hemodialysis-from arterial system to venous-dialysate bath and
semipermeable membrane.
Peritoneal dialysis-peritoneal cavity is the membrane for diffusion.
Always weigh the patient before dialysis.
Hemodialysis pump - dialysis fluid (dialysate) also can add med to
this if needed.
Access-Temporary (subclavian) until permanent is in place.

Permanent-cephalic/radial shunt.
Assess-Thrill-feel pulsing at site, will hear Bruit with stethoscope.
Problems with-fluid overload; electrolyte imbalance; anemia, infection, platelet abnormalities.

Peritoneal dialysis- measures what comes out. If 1500cc is put in, must get 1500 out- too much in will cause hypovolemic shock.
Peritoneal cavity, dwell, and remove
Types-continuous; intermittent
Advantages- Initiated more quickly- less stress and restrictions including dietary.
Disadvantages-Slower process; Infection

Transplantation-Most successful- Problem: Organ rejection.
Immunosuppression- avoid crowds
Close monitoring
Increased B/P, temp, pain at site
Increased BUN and creatinine
Fatigue, oliguria

Surgery/Cystectomy-removal of bladder
Urinary Diversion
Ileal conduit- 2 ureters/1stoma also can attach to sigmoid.
Pouch-Kock; Indiana- reservoir can cath themselves.
Urine breaks down to ammonia- 60%loss before symptoms, 90% loss will be in chronic renal failure.
Post op interventions
Monitor urine--mucous okay
Self-catheterization if needed
Teach proper bag care, how to, apply, empty when 1/2 full, odor.
Stressors
Inflammatory- Cystitis, Glomerulonephritis, and Pyelonephritis

Cystitis-Inflammation of bladder.
Painful urination, frequency, urgency, low back pain.
Treatment
Medication
Heat to area, Teach to urinate after sex.

Glomerulonephritis- always culture
Acute-streptococcal infection
Chronic-over years
Anasarca (total body edema, B/P, proteinuria, hypoalbuminemia-increased albumin-Protein is large molecule-loose protein will see in urine and is NOT normal.

Pyelonephritis-Bacteria from bladder- ascending bacteria.
Fever, chills, nausea and vomiting, flank pain.
Treatment-Antibiotics and antiseptics, fluid, rest, monitor urine.

Obstructions-hydronephrosis, stones, Cancer.
Hydronephrosis -Obstruction causing kidney to fill with fluid.
Acute-severe pain- uremia (itching)
Treatment-remove obstruction- Renal stones also can move to ureters. Send stones to lab.
Crystalloid or other substances.
Infection frequent
Low intake low fluids
Urinary stasis-sitting in bladder for long periods.
Prevention-increase fluids treat UTI, ID type of stone.

Renal stones-Flank pain, nausea and vomiting, blood in urine.
Treatment
-Increase fluids (to flush out), Analgesics, strain urine to find stones.
-Surgical Intervention- Lithotripsy (sound waves), nephro/pyelolithotomy when patient can't flush them out.

Cancer-Hematuria-usually late in disease
Treatment usually surgical removal, and or chemotherapy.

Causes of Urine Color
Antiseptics- urine color
Macrodantin-brown
Pyridium-orange
Sulfonamides- Bactrim/Septa- orange/red.
Prerenal failure caused by something, restriction in glomerulus filter rate. Intrarenal-disease in kidney. Post renal-after the kidney.

Renal Failure-acute reversible- 1/3 people can have problems and 5 percent will develop chronic renal failure.
Causes-infection, injury, inflammation, toxins, diabetes, hypertension.
Type-Acute Tubular Necrosis

Chronic Renal Failure
Causes-infection, inflammation, obstruction, systemic diseases.
-90 percent lost before symptoms
-inability to concentrate urine.
-uremia

Diagnosis
-renal biopsy, BUN and Creatinine -24 hour urine for creatinine
  Clearance.
-Uremia
-Hypertensive
-Skin-, scaly, yellow-gray color
-Anasarca- general body edema-tight/shiny and sometimes weeps
  Out of skin.
-Pruritus-itching
-Anemia
-Anorexia
-Uremic frost- indication of death looks like frost on body-waste
  Excretes through skin.

Labs
Hyperkalemia,
Hypocalcemia,
Hyperphosphatemia

Phases:
Insult phase-Oliguric-lots of urine output then decrease of urine,
vomiting, electrolyte imbalances, and edema.
Diuretic phase-take off extra fluid.
Recovery phase- low specific gravity, electrolytes back to normal.

Renal System Review
Excretory, metabolic, and regulatory processes.
Kidney Function
Regulation of body fluid volume and ion composition.
Removal of metabolic wastes and formation of urine.
Assistance in controlling acid-base.
Production of erythropoietin, RBC's
Regulation of blood pressure through fluid volume.
Production of active form of Vitamin D.
Elimination of drugs and toxins.

Macroscopic Structure
Functional renal tissues:
Cortex - outer portion, 1 cm deep.
Contains the glomerulus, or functional unit, extends downward into medulla.
Receives -90 percent of renal blood flow.

Functional Renal Tissues
Medulla - 5 cm deep
Contains tubule system, concentrates the filtrate (not urine yet)
Tubule system extends down in parallel from the cortex and is arranged into striated, fanlike masses called renal pyramids
Receives 10 percent of renal blood flow
Urine leaves through the papillae at ends.

Collection System
Urine flows from papillae into cuplike extensions, the minor and major calyx,
Then into the funnel-shaped dilation above the ureter - renal pelvis.
Pelvis and calyces can hold 3 - 5 ml urine.
Urine exits through ureters, into bladder, and is excreted through the urethra.

Innervation
Sympathetic (adrenergic) and parasympathetic (cholinergic)
Enter at the hilus. A denervated kidney will still form urine.
Transplanted kidneys are denervated, yet function normally.

Vascular Structures

Afferent arteriole (to the nephron) supplies blood to the glomerulus, under pressure.

Glomerulus (tuft of capillaries) is semipermeable.

Fluid and particles from blood (glomerular filtrate) pass into Bowman's capsule (part of tubular system).

Rest of blood flows out of glomerulus thru efferent (away) arteriole.

Glomerular capillaries are like the arterial end of tissue capillaries - where fluid and solutes leave.

After blood flows out of efferent arteriole, it circulates thru, a second, low pressure bed forming the Peritubular capillary network.

Peritubular Capillary Network

Like venous capillaries, they allow for exchange and reabsorption of fluid and solutes from tubular system.

Blood flows into interlobular vein and into inferior vena cava.

Tubular Structures

Bowman's capsule - cuplike structure that mostly surrounds the glomerulus and collects the filtrate (not called urine yet)

Filtrate flows into the tubule system to undergo exchanges and concentration.

Proximal (convoluted) tubule - short, coiled.

Loop of Henle - hairpin-like, descending limb dips into medulla, ascending loop cortex.

Ascending loop of Henle is attached to coiled distal (convoluted) tubule in cortex.

Empties unto collecting duct (tubule), joins others to form larger ducts and finally drains into the Pelvis through papillary ducts.

Glomerular Filtration Rate

GFR - amount of glomerular filtrate formed per minute.

Normal 90 - 125 ml/min (180 L/day)

Fluid part of the filtrate is renal plasma.

99 percent of filtrate is reabsorbed by tubules.

1 percent excreted as urine, 1.25 ml/min, 75 ml/hr or 1,800 ml/day.

Glomerular Hydrostatic Pressure-Controlled by changes in vasoconstriction of afferent and efferent arterioles.
Autoregulation - Constriction of afferent decreases blood flow and pressure in glomerulus, so decreases GFR.
Constriction of efferent increases pressure (afterload) so more filtrate enters Bowman's 30 Colloid Oncotic (Osmotic) Pressure.
Maintained by blood proteins, pulls fluid into capillary, or opposes the glomerular hydrostatic pressure.

Bowman's Hydrostatic Pressure
Small hydrostatic pressure that opposes the glomerular filtration. Increases in urinary obstruction or severe inflammation. Will stop GF if exceeds the glomerular pressure.

Tubular Reabsorption and Secretion
The other 2 forces in the formation of urine.
Glomerular filtrate in Bowman's contains much water, electrolytes, valuable solutes that need to be reabsorbed back into blood. Active transport, diffusion, osmosis used to reabsorb back into Peritubular capillaries.
Glucose, amino acids, vitamins and albumin normally totally reabsorbed (so not in the urine)

Tubular Secretion
Some substances secreted from peritubular capillaries into tubules to be excreted.
Important in H+ and K+, some drug excretion (penicillin)
Large amounts of Na+, Cl-, Ca+, Mg+, and PO4 are reabsorbed back into blood.

Functions of Tubular Sections
Proximal Tubule - 65% of Na+ and H2O are actively reabsorbed back into capillaries.
Loop of Henle:
Distal Tubule - lst part relatively impermeable to water. Affected by aldosterone, regulates the Na+ and K+ reabsorption.
H+ and HCO3- either secreted into tubule or reabsorbed into blood here. Ammonium ions secreted.

Collecting Tubule

Final site of concentration or dilution of urine.
Receives only 9.3 percent of original GF (12ml/min).
Fluid reabsorption controlled by ADH, causes the collecting tubule
to become highly permeable to H2O.
Makes urine more concentrated.

Regulation of Electrolytes

Na+ - affected by renal blood flow, GFR, tubular concentration of
Na+, presence of aldosterone.
Renal Hypoperfusion - more Na+ reabsorbed.
Renal Hyperperfusion - (osmotic diuresis, or increased water intake),
both Na+ and H2O.
Reabsorption is restricted (so more excreted.)

Na+ Regulation

Atrial natruretic hormone (ANH), beta natruretic peptide (BNP)
ventricles.
Released by heart when R atrial and ventricular pressures are
increased. Stimulate increased GFR
And Na+ and H20 excretion.

Regulation of Potassium

Affected by K+ intake, acid-base, aldosterone (increases excretion).
Normally increased dietary intake will be secreted by distal tubule.
Renal impairment - unable to secrete K+ normally, hyperkalemia.

Potassium

Metabolic and resp. alkalosis stimulate renal excretion of K+
(hypokalemia)
Metabolic and resp. acidosis depress excretion of K+ (hyperkalemia),
because excreting H+ ions.
Hyperkalemia stimulates aldosterone production to excrete K+,
retain Na+
Hypokalemia decreases aldosterone production.

Other Factors Influencing K+

Increase potassium excretion - potassium-losing diuretics (loop, Thiazide diuretics, and mannitol - osmotic diuretic)
Decrease K+ excretion - aldosterone deficiency and potassium-sparing diuretics.

Regulation of Acid-Base

Body fluids become acidic because of continuous production of strong acids.
Cellular metabolism byproducts are H+, carbonic, sulfuric, and phosphoric acids.

Renal Regulation of Acid-Base

Renal corrections are slower effective in excreting strong nonvolatile acids and excess alkali.
In acidosis, H+ ions excreted by tubules.
Kidney's primary mechanism for regulating acid-base (Na & HCO3 retained, H+ excreted as H2O, and ammonia)
Alkalosis - H+ retained, HCO3 excreted.
Renal Excretion of Metabolites
Excretes urea in tubules (nitrogenous waste products, like ammonia, converted to urea in liver)
Creatinine - waste product of muscle metabolism. Amount excreted is in proportion to muscle mass and renal function.
Enters glomerulus, not reabsorbed
Uric Acid - Product of dietary and endogenous amino acid metabolism

Renin

Juxtaglomerular apparatus - specialized group of cell in each nephron.
Formed by Juxtaglomerular cells of afferent arteriole and epithelial cells in distal tubule, macula densa.
Respond to decreases in tubular fluid flow and Na+ concentration.
Renin-angiotensin-aldosterone mechanism.

Erythropoietin- Kidneys produce and/or release.
Hormone stimulates RBC production in bone marrow.
Hypoxia, anemia, decreased blood flow to kidneys stimulate release.

Prostaglandins
Renal prostaglandin E2 (PGE2) produced
Increases renal plasma flow, redistributes the blood flow within the kidney, stimulates salt and water excretion.
Causes vasodilation and counteracts angiotensin II.

Vitamin D-Active form of vitamin D is a hormone produced by kidneys (1, 25-DHCC or 1, 25 Dihydroxycholecalciferol). Promotes the intestinal absorption of calcium. Vitamin D is consumed (milk) Or produced by the skin (sunlight) changed in the liver, and converted to active form by kidneys.
Without active Vitamin D, Ca+ not absorbed but lost in stool.
Insulin:
20 percent of insulin produced is catabolized in kidneys.
Less insulin required in chronic renal failure.

Gastrin-Hormone secreted by mucosa of the stomach. Causes gastric secretion of pepsin and HCL.
Normally degraded by kidneys.
Renal failure - high serum gastrin levels because hormone not degraded.
Increased risk of gastric ulcers.

Urine Collection Highlights
UA-Urinalysis - 1st voided urine in the am. Is best, more concentrated, more formed elements.
Need to clean peri- area first. Indicate if woman is menstruating.
Should go right to lab (less than 30 min)
Clean Catch Midstream-for C & S in non-cath pt. Clean, rinse peri-area. Start stream, and then catch urine. Need at least 10 cc.

Urine Collection
C & S-culture and sensitivity-from cath-use 10 cc syringe put in sterile collection cup. 24 hr urine-Get container from lab. May need to keep cool (basin or bucket of ice on floor). Have patient empty bladder, and then begin the 24 period. Instruct pt, tape on toilet, give commode, note on Foley bag. End with void or empty Foley 24 hrs later.

Abnormal Urine

Red or brownish (tea colored)-blood.
Yellow to green-brown-bile pigments.
Orange-drugs (Pyridium, Azulfidine, cascara), pigments, vegetables high in riboflavin (beets)
Sweet, fruity smell-acetone, dehydration, DM, fasting. Foul odor, cloudiness – infection.

Urine Lab Normal's

Bacteria < 1 – 2 per high powered field.
RBCs < 0 – 4 per hpf
WBC< 0 – 5 per hpf
Crystals - Few may be present, little clinical significance.
Casts - Few hyaline casts (mixture of mucus and congealed tubule globulin) normal.

Urine Lab Abnormal

RBCs-bleeding in kidneys or urinary tract (or contaminated with menstrual blood)
RBCs and casts (formed elements in the urine)-bleeding or infection in kidney.
No casts-bleeding in lower tract.
Casts-from WBCs, epithelial cells, protein from renal tubule.
Indicates renal tubular disorder.

Urine pH

Normal 4.5-8.0
Acidic with metabolic acidosis (DKA), recent ingestion of high protein foods.
Alkaline with metabolic alkalosis (vomiting, sodium bicarb)
Low protein foods (vegetables), or urea splitting bacteria (Proteus mirabilis)

Specific Gravity

Measures concentration of solutes in urine.
Normal 1.001-1.030
The more concentrated, the higher the SG
Urine osmolality more accurate guide.

Abnormal in Urine

Protein – normally none (0 – 18 mg/dl). Albumin in urine indicates renal disease.
Can lose up to 20 gms/day.
Glucose – normally none (until blood glucose more than 160 – 200). May be from DM, or TPN.
Acetone – ketones, produced by cells burning fat (DKA, fever, starvation, diarrhea, prolonged vomiting, anesthesia)

Blood Urea Nitrogen

Normal 10 – 30 mg/dL
Increase reflects protein breakdown (increase in dietary, muscle breakdown, sepsis
Fevers, dehydration, shock, CHF, GI bleed excessive exercise.
Renal insufficiency

Increased BUN

During dehydration, renal tubules increase reabsorption of water, as well as reabsorption of urea.
Increases BUN. In renal failure, BUN increases because the glomeruli cannot filter it.
Decreased BUN, Overhydration
Malnutrition (less protein to break down)
Severe liver disease (can't convert ammonia to urea)

Creatinine

Normal 0.5 – 1.5 mg/dL
Enzyme in skeletal muscle, part of muscle contraction physiology.
Constant in relation to muscle mass. Completely excreted, not reabsorbed in renal tubules.
Not influenced by dietary intake, or dehydration.
More sensitive indicator of renal dysfunction is increased,
Elevation consistent with 50% nephron loss.
Decrease can be seen in elderly or conditions with decreased muscle mass.

BUN/Creatinine Ratio
Can't just look at BUN to evaluate renal function or treatment.
Normal ratio of BUN: Creatinine 10:1 to 15:1
Increased ratio (elevated BUN) – dehydration, protein breakdown.
Decreased ratio (decreased BUN) – low protein, overhydration, liver failure.
Normal ratio, with both elevated – renal failure.

Renal Biopsy
Long needle used to obtain small tissue sample. Local anesthesia, fluoroscopy. Examines the structure of glomeruli, monitor progression of chronic renal disease, dx clot, stone, or tumor. High risk for bleeding.

Post Renal Biopsy
Lie still for 4 hrs, sandbag on site.
Bed rest 24 hrs. To prevent bleeding.
No strenuous activities for several days.
Report burning urination, flank pain, dizziness, hematuria, infection signs.
Acute Renal Failure (ARF)
Rapid deterioration
Accumulation of nitrogenous wastes in blood - uremia or azotemia (BUN, creatinine)
Sudden inability of the kidney to regulate H_2O and electrolytes.
Can develop over hrs, days, or weeks.
May be reversible or lead to irreversible chronic renal failure.
Actual damage occurs to renal tissue. (25%)
GFR not improved immediately after removing cause.
Tubular damage -ATN
Renal disease, hypoperfusion, nephrotoxin.

Incidence and Epidemiology
Caused by: Ischemia to kidney.
Nephrotoxic agents - drugs, contrast dyes, heavy metals.
Inflammatory processes – acute pyelonephritis, glomerulonephritis (streptococcus)
Systemic, vascular disorders. Pregnancy disorders.

Acute Tubular Necrosis

Most common causes: ischemia.
May occur after few minutes or hrs of hypotension.
At risk if MAP < 70 mmHg.
Causes vasoconstriction and decreased GFR.
Tubular dysfunction develops.
Nephrotoxin - cause direct injury to tubule cells.
NSAIDS may contribute (block vasodilating prostaglandins)

Pathophysiology

Interstitial edema causes compression, and casts, debris cause tubular lumen occlusion. Leads to necrosis, degeneration of tubular epithelium – oliguria. Glomerular filtrate may be reabsorbed due to altered glomerular permeability, vasoconstriction, and tubular necrosis. Total renal blood flow decreased by 50%
Clinical Findings
Oliguria, sometimes anuria (unlike CRF) in 1 - 7 days.
More acutely ill, less time to adjust to uremia
Well defined stages:
Onset, oliguric-anuric, diuretic, convalescent.

Stages of ARF

Onset:
Usually abrupt, begins with precipitating event hours, days before.
Oliguric-Anuric Stage - u/o < 400/24 hrs
May appear within 72 hrs, acute uremia. Lasts 7 - 14 days to weeks.
Healing begins within 48 hrs, but impairment persists.
The longer the oliguria, the poorer the prognosis.
May have normal u/o, but increased BUN/creatinine, signs of uremia (nonoliguric acute renal failure).

Oliguric Stage – increased BUN, creatinine, K+, PO4, Mg+, decreased creatinine clearance (urine).
Decreased pH (acidosis), HCO3-, Ca+, Hct (dilutional), Hgb (erythropoietin). UA – decreased volume, mild to mod proteinuria, casts, cellular debris, red and white blood cells, increased specific gravity.

Diuretic Stage - High output failure.
U/O- urine output > 500/ 24 hrs.
BUN stabilizes, begins to decrease
Tubules healing, can excrete wastes, but can't concentrate filtrate.
May last 1 – 3 wks. Monitor for hypovolemia, decreased Na+,
decreased K+
Diagnostic Studies   Diuretic Stage.
BUN, creatinine slowly decreases.
May become hypokalemic, develop metabolic alkalosis.

Convalescent stage - BUN stable, normal activity.
Several months to year for complete recovery (may never get back to
baseline Treatment.
Treat underlying cause
Prevent progression to permanent ARF and Identify serious
complications. Promote comfort, relief of uremic symptoms.

End Stage Renal Disease ESRD
Substantial reduction of GFR that develops over years/decades (< 5-
10 percent of normal)
Creatinine clearance <5-10 ml/min.
Results in permanent kidney damage.
May lose up to 80 percent of function before diagnosing.
CRF progresses to ESRD - dialysis and/or transplant necessary to
sustain life.

ESRD Risk Factors
Diabetes, Hypertension
Glomerulonephritis (Inflammatory process of glomerulus)
Cystic kidney diseases

Fluid Overload
Hypervolemia (HTN, increased Na+, CHF)
Fluid restriction 1,000 – 1,500 ml (pre-dialysis U/O + 500-600 ml)
Daily wt (less than 1-1.5 kg between runs)
Monitor lung sounds, peripheral and dependent edema.
Measure frozen liquids, syrups/water.

Electrolytes – Na+

Hyper or hyponatremia (depending on amount of free water retained)
Usually hypernatremic – restrict Na+ to 2 – 3 gms/a day, to prevent H2O retention.
Cannot use salt substitutes because of KCL
Season food with lemon, garlic, vinegar.

Electrolytes – K+

Hyperkalemia more than 5.5 head ache, abdominal, pain, tachypnea, weakness, nausea, vomiting, malaise, acidosis
EKG – peaked T wave, prolonged PR, wide QRS, ventricular tachycardia, asystole
Restrict to 2- 3 gms/day.
Kayexalate- oral, enema. Exchanges Na+ for K+, binds with K+ in gut and is excreted in the stool.

Hyperkalemia

Insulin and D50 IVP will push K+ back into the cells, temporarily.
HCO3 – corrects acidosis temporarily so K+ returns to cells.
Calcium gluconate IV – reverses cardiotoxic effects of hyperkalemia and prevents arrest.
K+ restricted diet 2 - 3 gms (40 mEq)

Nutritional Guidelines

Protein, Na, K, PO4 and fluids are controlled to meet each patient's needs. Protein sources should be of high biologic value.
High Na and high K foods should be avoided.
Sufficient calories and nutrients are provided to meet daily requirements.

Dialysis Goals:

Remove excess protein metabolism end products from blood (urea, creatinine). Maintain safe concentrations of serum electrolytes (K+)
Remove excess body fluid. Correct acidosis by adding HCO3

How It Works -Utilizes principles of diffusion and osmosis
-Dialysate solution (concentration ordered by Dr) containing varying
   amounts of electrolytes, dextrose, bicarbonate.
-The dialysate is on one side of the semipermeable membrane, blood
   on the other.

Diffusion

-Solutes move from area of higher to lower concentration. So excess
   electrolytes (K+, MG+) and waste solutes move from the blood
   into the dialysate (to be discarded).
-Dialysate will contain electrolytes that we don't want to remove

   (Na+ and Cl- isotonic, CA+ added).
-HCO3 or lactate (used to make HCO3) added to enter blood and
   buffer acidosis.

Osmosis

-Movement of water molecules from area of higher to lower
   concentration.
-Glucose and dextrose added to dialysate to act as osmotic gradient.
   More solutes and less water in the dialysate, so water moves out of
   blood.
-Hemodialysis machines can also create a pressure gradient to "pull"
   more fluid off.
-Increased temperature, rate of blood flow and time of contact will
   also increase solute and water exchange.

Dialysate Concentrations

-The higher the concentrations will still exchange solutes, but more
   water is pulled (4.25%) (Decrease in Blood pressure).
-The lower concentrations increase solute exchange, less water loss
   (1.5 %, 2.5%). Use with decreased BP, may alternate solutions.

Hemodialysis

-Blood removed through an access device, pumped through a
   machine (warmed, heparinized) and through tiny capillary tubes
   (semipermeable membranes).

The blood exchanges solutes and water with the dialysate bath surrounding all the "capillaries" and return to the body. 250-500 ml pulled and returned per min. -Process repeated for 3-4 hrs.

Arteriovenous Access
-Hemo stick- temporary for fast access.
-Perma Cath – permanent double lumen catheter. Double lumen catheter placed in subclavian or jugular vein. Inserted by radiologist.
-Blood pulled from one lumen, and returned through the other.
-More long term access is achieved through surgically created AV fistula or graft. Temporary cath used until these are healed.

Internal Vascular Accesses
-AV fistula-surgical anastomosis of an artery and vein (usually forearm). Takes 4-6 weeks to heal.
-AV graft-If the artery and vein are too small to join together (Diabetics with atherosclerosis), an artificial, flexible tube is anastomosed to an artery, the other end to a vein.

After the Dialysis
-Vital signs, weight (calculate wt loss)
-Monitor access site for patency, bleeding, and any generalized bleeding.
-Administer late meds per doctor's orders.
-Let the pt rest-will be extremely tired. Dialysis is exhausting.

Peritoneal Dialysis **PD**
-Works by same principles as hemodialysis.
-Fluid is instilled into the peritoneal cavity via a surgically placed catheter, with many openings. The dialysate exchanges with blood in capillaries in the peritoneum (semipermeable membrane)

Candidates for PD
-Pts that can't tolerate the heparin with hemodialysis, or BP too low with rapid fluid loss.
-Vascular access problems

-Patients who want to do the dialysis at home, avoid coming to hemodialysis 3 times/week. More effective than HD, more mobility, fewer dietary restrictions.
-Need to be able to learn, manage sterile technique, and have room for large volume of supplies (many liter bags) Time consuming.

Contraindications for PD

-Recent abdominal surgery, paralytic ileus, bowel distension, abdominal adhesions, opens draining wound (high risk for infection), obesity, recurrent hernias, chronic back pain, COPD.
-Hypoproteinemia- some protein is lost in the dialysate solution. Need more protein in diet.
-Not the treatment for rapid correction of imbalances or acidosis, takes longer to correct.

Continuous Ambulatory Peritoneal Dialysis. CAPD.

New dialysate is instilled and allowed to dwell in the peritoneal cavity until next exchange (4hrs). Dialysate is drained into a bag, below level of patient (drain time 20-30 min). Patient has more freedom, until the next time (4-10 hrs). No machinery needed, more liberal protein, fluid intake. Can travel with bags.

Nephrotic Syndrome Child

(Nephrosis or glomerulo-nephritis). Condition of kidneys that have marked amounts of protein in the urine.
Idiopathic Nephrosis – cause is seldom determined.
Most common type seen in early childhood. Glomeruli becomes damaged, allows albumin & protein to enter the urine.
Decreased serum protein (hypoproteinemia)
Increased serum cholesterol (hyperlipidemia)
More common in boys than girls.
Most often seen between 2 & 7 years of age.
Prognosis good – usually outgrow problem.
Other types may develop renal failure & require dialysis or transplantation.

S&S
Primary sign is edema
First around eyes and ankles
Generalized (child not sick)
Marked increased wt. 2nd to fluid retention.
Abdominal distention
Pale, irritable, listless with poor appetite.
Urine dark & frothy, output decreased.
May have diarrhea and vomiting.
UA = massive albumin (protein)

Treatment
Renal biopsy
Renal Ultra Sound
Steroids (prednisone) induce diuresis.
For 1-2 months
No immunizations
Diuretics are not effective in reducing nephrotic edema.
Urine must be free of protein for 5 days.
Then check every other day for 3 to 6 months.

Nursing Care
Weight child same time on same scale daily.
Measure abdominal girth every day.
Well balanced diet with no added salt while edema present.
Small frequent meals – favorite foods when possible.
Strict I & O (pt. Education is. very important) 1g equals 1ml
Urine color, odor, quantity.
Daily urine specific gravity & protein.
Skin care, positioning
Infection control (esp. if on steroids)
Emotional support
Frequent repositioning to prevent skin breakdown.
Urinary Tract Infection (UTI)
More common in girls than boys
Urethra is shorter & closer to anus
Retention of urine/vaginitis
Avoid nylon underwear & bubble baths

Infant
Fever, weight loss, failure to thrive, nausea and vomiting, increased voiding.
Older child
Urinary frequency, painful micturition, onset of bed wetting, abdominal pain, hematuria.
Nursing Care: urine collection, I & O.
Patient/parent education.
Proper cleansing of perineal area.

Wilms Tumor
Nephroblastoma – kidney bud tumor.
Compresses kidney usually encapsulated.
Seldom affects both kidneys.
Most common malignancies of early life.
Thought to have genetic base.
Usually discovered before 3 yrs of age.
Large mass in the abdomen.

Treatment: surgery (extensive incision), chemotherapy & radiation.
Parent Education
Avoid unnecessary handling of abdomen.

Acute Glomerulonephritis
Thought to be an antigen-antibody reaction caused by group A beta hemolytic strep infection.
Occurs 1 to 3 weeks after strep infection.
S&S
Gross hematuria, oliguria, edema, and proteinuria.
Smoky brown urine from RBCs.
Most patients Recover fully in 1 to 3 months.
Treatment: Restriction of dietary sodium & fluid based on HTN edema.
Restrict foods high in potassium – during episodes of oliguria.
Nursing Care
Accurate I & O, Monitor Vital Signs, Observe for fatigue, Prevent Chilling, Limit activity until gross hematuria subsides. Prone to HTN – any changes notify physician immediately can have surgery.

Hypospadias

Congenital defect – urinary meatus is below the tip of the penis.
May be accompanied by chordee (downward curvature of the penis caused by a fibrotic band of tissue.
Circumcision by reconstructive urologist.

Epispadias

Opening of the urinary meatus on the upper surface of the penis.
Fairly uncommon. Requires surgical intervention.
Separation/Mutilation issues for child.

Hydrocele

Collection of fluid into the scrotum when the processus vaginalis (skin fold) doesn't fuse separating the peritoneal cavity from the scrotum. Corrects itself by 1 year of age – surgery is indicated if not.

Phimosis

Unretractable foreskin. May not be detected until 3 months
Treatment only if hinders urination.
If possible stretch back prepuce to expose the urethral opening.

Paraphimosis

Foreskin is retracted over the glans and fixed.
Causes constriction and decreased blood flow.
Treatment: surgical intervention.

Cryptorchidism

Undescended testes
Unknown cause
Continue to secrete hormones.
2nd sex characteristics unaffected.
If bilat – may have sterility
Descends about 1 yr of age
If not: Orchiopexy (fixation of testes)
Nursing care: Parent/patient education.
What they know & understand.
Discuss fears of homosexuality.

Chapter 5

Nervous System

Anatomy Review
Upper Motor Neurons, neurons in the brain, spinal cord.
Lower Motor Neurons, Nerves outside the spinal cord and in periphery.

Impulse Conduction
Afferent fibers - bring sensory information to the neuron cell body or CNS.
Efferent fibers - bring motor impulse from the neuron, out of CNS to peripheral tissues.
Short dendrites (afferent) bring impulse to cell body. Resting membrane is + outside, inside.
Impulses travel faster through myelinated (white - insulated) axons.
Electricity jumps from one node of Ranvier to next.
Electrical Depolarization
Electrical impulse changes membrane charges (now - outside, + inside). K+ leaves cell, Na+ enters. Impulse spreads down long axon, neurotransmitters are released.
Electrolytes reversed by ion pumps (requires ATP), so cell is ready for next depolarization.

Neurotransmitters
Released into synaptic cleft, from storage in vesicles.
They will continue to act on the neurons, so they need to stop by.
Taken back up by the vesicle
Degraded by enzymes
Diffusion out of the synapse

Chief Neurotransmitters:
Parasympathetic: Nervous System
Acetylcholine (ACH) (also found in SNS).
Degraded in synapse by acetylcholinesterase.

Sympathetic: Nervous System, norepinephrine. Most taken back up by vesicle, some diffused or is, Broken down by monamine oxidase (MAO) (So, MAO inhibitors increase SNS activity, overdose).

Inhibitory Neurotransmitters:
GABA: gamma aminobutyric acid-Regulates available energy Inhibits brain, spinal, retinal functions. (Less GABA can contribute to seizure activity)
Dopamine: Controls fine movement (Parkinson's), sensory integration, emotional behavior.
Serotonin: Controls heat regulation, sleep, hunger, and behavior, sense of well being (chocolate!)
Excitatory Neurotransmitters
Substance P - released by pain fiber terminals in spinal cord, increasing perception of pain. Balanced by inhibitory encephalin and endorphins (involved with decreasing perception and emotions).

Patient History
1. Motor disturbances, deficits - weakness, uncoordinated, tremors, paresis (partial paralysis), paralysis.
2. Trouble writing, speaking or getting right words out, swallowing, problem with bowel or bladder control, sexual.
3 Seizures, lapses in attention, Sensory deviations - numbness, tingling, prickling, lack of feeling.
Normal sense of smell, vision changes or field decreases, hearing, dizziness. Coldness/warmth of feet and hands?
4. Altered states of consciousness - fainting, confusion, loss of memory.

Differentiating Between Neuro and Other Systems
Heart Stokes-Adams syncope- convulsions, unconsciousness from temporary ventricular slowing or standstill.
CV thrombi or emboli cause strokes, vessels rupture. Peripheral arterial ischemia.
Postural hypotension - dizziness, fainting.
Hematologic - pernicious or hemolytic anemia cause neuro changes (hypoxia)

Assessment of Consciousness and Mental State
Cognitive functioning-thinking ability.
Emotions
Personality and psychological status.
Physiologic changes

Assessing Cognitive Function
Describe observations in behavioral terms.
Attention span: repeat 7 digits
Orientation: time, place, others, self, general question knowledge (president)
Memory, concentration and past medical history.
Intellect: vocabulary, education, and work experience.
Flow of Speech: rhythm, pace, clarity.
Perception-answer appropriately, follows commands, dress, and moves appropriately.
Abstract thinking-proverbs.
Motor planning-complete tasks in sequence.
Calculation-count back from 100, by 7, by 2
Judgment-insight questions.
Appearance-clothing, hair, hygiene, teeth, nails.
Behavior-mobility, energy, recognition, tolerance of new situations.

Emotional Assessment
Anxiety, depression - sleep patterns, slowness in thought, speech, movement, restlessness, muscle tension.
Bowel disturbances, fatigue, loss of appetite/wt, menstruation, libido.
Mood-appropriate response for situation. Discussion of feelings (gloom, death wishes, suspicion, guilt, manic)

Assessing Personality and Psychological State
Personality/lifestyle before illness
Education, goals, work, hobbies, family relationships, sexual orientation, use of drugs and or alcohol.
Health care-Listen for delusions, illusions, hallucination
Motivation-ask patients plan for actions to improve their condition.

Glasgow Coma Scale
Level of consciousness 1st
Orientation
Pupil Response (PERLA)
Motor Response
Vital Signs
Reflexes
Cranial nerve assessment

Physiologic Changes - Vital Signs
Temp, pulses in extremities, RR and pattern
Signs of increased ICP:
Increased BP with widened pulse pressure.
Decreased RR

Cerebellar Tests
Romberg test: Stand with feet together with eyes open for 5 sec, then
with eyes closed for 5 sec. should be able to stand without swaying.
Eyes closed shouldn't affect. Deep knee bend, hop in place, walk heel
to toe, and normal gait-with eyes open. Patient in bed-run heel down
shin of opposite leg.

Sensory System
Anesthesia, hypoesthesia, hyperesthesia, pain.
Use light touch from distal to proximal.
Dysfunction involves dermatomes supplied by nerve plexus.

Sensory Assessment
Glove and stocking-distal symmetric neuropathy from DM-diabetes
melitis, alcoholic neuropathy. Use the point and hub of needle.
Extinction: touch opposite sides simultaneously,
Have patient identify sharp or dull, point to area touched (tactile
localization).
Two-point discrimination: can recognize 2 points 4-5 mm apart on
fingertips, most sensitive.
Vibration: tuning fork over joints, skin

Position sense - move thumb to different positions (patient identifies position)
Stereognosis: recognizes objects by touch.
Graphesthesia: recognizes writing on skin.
Identify textures and weights.
Deep pressure - squeeze Achilles tendon.

Cerebrospinal Fluid Analysis

Lumbar puncture (LP): large needle inserted into subarachnoid space between L-4 and L-5 spinal canal.
Spinal cord ends at L-2
Purpose: to measure CSF pressure, CSF analysis, inject a contrast medium for studies, drain off CSF.

LP-Lumbar Puncture

Contraindicated if signs of increased ICP are present.
Consent, sterile procedure at bedside.
Local anesthetic, spinal needle, CSF drips into opened test tubes.
Manometer on stopcock to measure pressure.
(60 -150 mm H2O nml)
CSF-Cerebral Spinal Fluid
Examined for protein, glucose, blood cell counts, culture for bacteria.

Terminology

Aphasia-speaking or understanding words / Receptive Aphasia -can't understand.
Expressive Aphasia-can't speak.
Dysphasia-speaking-can't speak clear.
Dysphagia-swallowing.
Atrophy-deterioration of muscle.
Ataxia-lack if order, coordination, irregular muscle movement.
Hemiplegia-paralysis (feeling) on one side of the body.
Hemiparesis-weakness on one side of body.
Paraplegia-below T1-lower part of body.
Quadriplegia-above T1 loss to all extremities.
C5- increases death- respiratory (phrenic nerve)

Sensory and Neurologic Conditions

Otitis Media-Inflammation & buildup of fluid after a bacterial or viral invasion.

Secretory otitis media-(SOM)-moisture or water in ear

Acute serous otitis media-(ASOM)-fluid buildup, feel a lot of pressure.

Acute purulent otitis media-eardrum ruptures gets hole in ear and drains pus.

Chronic otitis media- middle ear infection, remove tonsils sometimes.

Signs & Symptoms-Otitis Media

Acute, stabbing pain in the ear-prolonged crying while rubbing or tugging at the ear.

Some bleeding or discharge of pus from ear-most likely occurs if eardrum ruptures to relieve pressure from the fluid.

Fever, Nausea & vomiting; especially young child-Temporary hearing loss.

Cerebral Palsy-group of disorders affects the motor centers of the brain, causing problems with movement and coordination.

Does not impair the thinking process.

Causes: Congenital problems involving the CNS.

Decreased oxygen to infant during pregnancy.

Exposure during pregnancy to toxins or infections.

Premature births

Head injuries, meningitis & encephalitis.

Sometimes no known cause.

S&S Varying with each child-Range from mild to severe.

Mental retardation sometimes-most have normal intelligence.

Cues: Agar's scores <5 at 1 minute.

Seizures 1st 48 hours of life.

Delayed achievements of milestones- know what is normal.

Increased muscle tone-abnormal reflexes. Spasticity: tension in certain muscle groups.

Dyskinetic: involuntary purposeful movements that interfere with normal motion facial, eyes, also can have seizures.

Ataxia: lack of muscle coordination- mostly emotional.

Medical Treatment
Highly individualistic depending on the severity.
Physical/occupational therapy.
Surgery for deformities (sometimes)
Special & communication devices.
High caloric diets- because of nonstop movement.

Treatment Protocol of Cerebral Palsy
Establish-communication, Optimize existing muscles.
Provide intellectual stimulation, Socialization.
Provide technology and encourage self care.
Provide multidisciplinary help.

Interventions
Prevent the formation of contractures-What you don't use you lose.
Opportunity to play
Parent education
Frequent naps/quiet room-Treat like other kids their age don't want
pity accept them for who they are.

Epilepsy-Recurrent seizure disorder-some treat for short time others
lifetime.
Paroxysmal attacks of unconsciousness or impaired consciousness
Febrile Seizures <102 are not Epilepsy
Postictal State-dazed confused-sleep for a while.
Status Epilepticus-series of convulsion from abrupt withdrawal of
medication.
Nonconvulsive seizures-repetitive behavior-loss of muscle tone.
Treatment-Protect from harm-Anticonvulsive Medication.
Ketogenic diet has calming effect- high protein low carbohydrates.

Tests:-Lumbar Puncture/Spinal Tap
Purpose-Assess pressure (nl 50-175mmH2O) Inject medication-
placed in the subarachnoid space, (3rd Lumbar) or around there.
Obtain fluid for analysis- for infections and CNS disorders, use a
small bore needle.

Nursing Implications Head flexed on chest, knees up to abdomen-
Encourage PO fluids
Flat in bed 6-8 hrs- prevent HA, takes that long for CSF to replace.
Blood Plug- prevents leakage, if they use the plug patient is out in less
time 2 hrs approx.
Looking for blood glucose and protein fluid pressure 50/175 fill 3
tubes label 1, 2, 3, Blood in tubes 2 and 3 are not acceptable.

EEG-electroencephalography-they do 3 tests to determine brain
dead, pupils are fixed and dilated.
Purpose -Assess electrical activity of brain cells, not evasive.
Electrodes placed on head signals generated by neurons by surface of
cerebral cortex, excellent test for seizures.

Nursing Implications
Wash hair before (so patches will stay) and after (wash out glue from
electrodes). Must be very quiet while test is running, if anything is
running in the room it must be recorded as noise.

EMG-electromyography-signature-NPO-painful procedure.
Purpose Assess electrical activity of skeletal muscle/response to
peripheral motor and sensory nerves to electrical stimuli.
Diagnosing neuromuscular disorders recorded on an oscilloscope.

Nursing Implications-Hold meds relaxants, cholinergic, and
anticholinergics, no smoking or caffeine, tell patient it is an
uncomfortable procedure.
Cholinergic (smooth)-Anticholinergenic (skeletal)

Myelogram-NPO 8 hrs prior-inject dye-invasive (In Back)
Purpose Lesions, disc problems, tumors.
Nursing Implications-Assess for allergy to iodine or shellfish tell
patient will feel Warm flush when dye injected.
Post procedure assess pulses and sensation in extremities, Monitor
for voiding-coccyx area control urination,
Neuro check distal to injection site.

Angiography

NPO 8 hrs prior-inject dye-and invasive into (Femoral Artery)
Purpose-Visualize cerebral arteries.
Nursing Implications-Allergy to iodine and shellfish-tell will feel
Warm Flush as dye inject.
-Post procedure-monitor for bleed at site, dysphagia (swallowing) and
  respiratory distress.
*MRI measurement of blood flow

Assessment

Speech, behavior, coordination, alertness, comprehension
History-genetic disorders, how long, loss of consciousness,
difficult speak, head injury, infections of EENT, black outs.
Paraesthesia (numb tingling).

Physical

Coordination and Balance
(Romberg /close eyes) feet together arms at side.
Strength-0-5 scale 0=no movement.
Weak
Moves when supported against gravity.-Active muscles movement
against gravity.
Full ROM against gravity some weakness w/ resistance.-Full ROM
against gravity and resistance.

Gait-posture

Reflexes-swallowing, gag, feel throat (no fluid)
knee jerk when hit patella.
Clonus- repetitive movement after dorsal flex.
Babinski- +normal in newborn not in adults-shows inter cranial
pressure in adults if toes fan out.
Normal adults curl down.
Doll's Eyes--intracranial pressure- normal when head turns eyes
follow few seconds later.

Mental Functioning
Neuro check
Glasgow scale less than 7-coma-15 normal, decorticate-abnormal
flex-towards medial /decerebrate-abnormal extension-away from
medial
Vital Signs
Pupil reaction-normal is symmetrical, asymmetrical means opposite
side of brain problems, use pen light outside in, finger out to in, give
no meds as masks the problems narcotics (pinpoint pupils)
Motor function

Nursing Diagnosis Ineffective breathing, Impaired physical
mobility, Self-care deficit, Ineffective family coping.

Common Problem
Dysphagia- set in semi fowlers before/after eating or drinking;
Sit all patients at same table with dysphasia so keep eye on them.
Incontinence-train bladder, clamp off bag to see what patient. Can do
to eliminate, bowel training can use fiber, fluid.
Pain
Confusion-safety is a factor, calm, distracters
 Avoids restrains at all cost.
Aphasia
Sexual dysfunction-don't need sex to be sensual.
Psychosocial concerns-ability to work and family situations.

Stressors
IICP-Infectious, diseases, Head Injuries, Intracranial tumor, Cerebral
Vascular, Accident, Epilepsy,
Trigeminal neuralgia, Spinal cord injury. Parkinsonism, Multiple
Sclerosis, Alzheimer's, Myasthenia Gravis.

Cranial Nerves12 nerves
Not only assessing function of nerve but function of brain stem,
depending on where the nerve originates.

Cranial Nerves-

1	2	3	4	5	6	7	8	9
10	11	12						

ON OCCASION OUR TRUSTY TRUCK   ACTS   FUNNY, Very   GOOD   VECHICLE   ANY   HOW
  Olfac   Optic   Ocular   Troc   Trigem-   Abduc   Facial   Vestib   Glossoph   Vagus   Asses Hypogloss

I-Olfactory

II-Optic

III-Oculomotor

IV-Trochlear

V-Trigeminal

VI-Abducens

VII-Facial

VIII-Vestibulocochlear- acoustic

IX-Glossopharyngeal

X-Vagus

XI-Accessory

XII-Hypoglossal

Increased Intracranial Pressure
S & S-Increased B/P, Lethargy, Decreasing consciousness, slowing of speech, Delay in responses,
Treatment suggests.
Osmotic diuretics (Mannitol) cross the blood brain barriers; Use filter needle- mannitol crystallizes in the tubing.
Decadron- steroid, for inflammation-less inter cranial pressure.
Barbiturates-Phenobarbital want to slow things down, slowing down decreases ICP.
Keep slightly dehydrated.
IV TKO- use large bore needle number 18

Check

1 consciousness

2 pupils number 3 ocular motor if full blown and fixed (late sign of trouble)

3 motor, sensory function muscles.

4 VS - (Cushing's triad) - wide pulse pressure, irregular respirations, bradycardia= ICP

Raise bed no more than 30°

Contra lateral-opposite side of injury.

Kernig's sign-flex hip 90°, and then extend knee movement produces pain in hamstring.

Brudzinski sign- when flex patient neck, hips flex.

Meningitis

Inflammation of membranes (meninges) covering the brain and spinal cord, Results from bacteria or virus passing the blood brain barrier and infecting the CSF.

S & S- -Severe persistent head ache > with head shakings- Photophobia-light sensitive. Increase irritability, delirium. Nuchal rigidity-stiff neck is the classic sign, exaggerated deep tendon reflexes. Seizures may be present, nausea and vomiting. Lethargy, fever and or convulsions.

Nursing Interventions:

Assess for ICP, Look for Herpes simplex.

Room quiet and dim lights, Monitor I & O.

Assess bowel sounds and for stool softness Minimal amount with enema (increases ICP).

Diagnosis/Treatment

Blood Cultures, Lumbar puncture -CSF Cultures.

IV antibiotics - broad spectrum then specific.

Isolation- because contagious.

Vital Signs, Neurologic assessment

Intake & Output

Dimly lit room-Keep noise to a minimum-

Disturb as little as possible.

Gillian-Barré Syndrome

Unknown cause - Pathology-demyelization (white coating on myelin sheath)

Autoimmune response destroys myelin sheath.

Inflammation, edema and nerve root compression follows viral infection or gastroenteritis.

S & S- Paresthesia - abnormal sensations, Pain, Progressive ascending paralysis, from feet up then paralyses respiratory/diaphragm, usually resolves itself.

Treatment-Supportive of family, Plasmapheresis to filter out the blood.

Interventions: Acute-sustain life, prevent complications, comfort, Static-preventing complications, Rehabilitation-can take up to 2 years.

Head Injury Terminology

Concussion-compression at site of blow trauma to head with no visual injury,

can loose consciousness <5 minutes, head ach, nausea and vomiting, amnesia.

Contusion-Bruised, broken blood vessels increased ICP.

Coup -not just place of impact countercoup- opposite side of impact. Need a baseline to go on.

1st signs are deterioration, restless, agitation, lethargy.

2nd sign labored irregular breathing, wide pulse pressure, and pupils.

Subdural Hematoma

S & S-Increasing ICP, 24hours ice, don't eat or exercise.

Can take weeks to show symptoms, head ache, Pupils, sluggish, project vomiting.

Treatment assess every 2 hours

Conservative-=decrease oral intake to try resolve itself.

Burr holes

Interventions-monitor for CSF leakage (halo or glucose) Serous outside, blood inside.

Test halo for glucose by dipstick.

Vital signs, head of bed to 30 degrees, cover draining with sterile dressing,

Teach not to blow or pick their nose =increase ICP.

Dura /Out-Arachnoid/Mid- CSF in this space, Pia/Inner.
Look for drainage from ears and nares.
Periorbital edema-swelling eyes.
Post auricle ecchymosis-discoloration around ears.
Subdural tear veins that drain brain and accumulate beneath the Dura.
Epidural- arterial bleed between Skull and Dura.
Acute Subdural- w/in 24 hrs
Subacute more than 24 hours less than week.
Chronic Subdural- low impact injury shows up weeks or months later.

Intracranial Tumors
*72 hours after surgery critical due to fluid influx- maybe death.
S & S- Frequently benign but still serious.
Treatment-Radiation, chemotherapy, immunotherapy, surgery
Curative/Palliative.
Nurse: Monitor ICP and blood pressure.

Cerebral Vascular Accident
Stroke more in Males and Doubles each decade after 55.
Tissue Plasminogen- 3 hours onset of stroke.
Thrombolytic w/in6 hours of stroke "activase-tpn.
First 6 hours of stroke damage is done. Timing is everything +6 weeks to rehab to get back what they can.

Surgical Carotid Endarterectomy- if 100%concluded can't do anything.
Different kinds of plaque- some break off, some stay solid.
Prevention Manage risk factors;-Risk factors-stop smoking keep blood pressure down.
Keep blood sugar stable.

S & S: TIA-transient ischemic attack, interruption of the blood flow to the brain.
Auscultate carotid artery to hear abnormal BRUIT sound (swishing).

Treatment for Carotid Endarterectomy
Treatment/Phase I must find out exact time of incident, count from last time they were ok.
Determine cause if not hemorrhagic: within 6 hours of onset: tPA (Activase).
Tissue plasminogen activator to dissolve blood clots.
After 6 -hours heparin in hospital convert to Coumadin= to prevent polycythemia (thick blood) PT /INR important.
Determine extent, GOALS
Establish baseline data
Preserve joint and muscle function. Prevent complications.

Phase II/Rehabilitation
Adequate airway, adequate nutrition, Finger foods, if swallow and chewing is good thicken liquids.
Effective communication-Strength muscles, TEDS, Self care.
Left Side- Slow behavior, Speech, Aphasia, Difficult directions.
Right Side-Impulsive, Short attention, emotional, Impulsive reactions.

Seizures
Hyperactive neurons use excessive O2 & Glucose, Jacksonian March-eyelid-same side motor area.
Causes-Epilepsy; high fever; ERSD=Irreversible state where kidney function is less than 10-15 percent.
Diagnosis by -EEG, MRI

Absence-petit mal- Daydreaming Lasts few seconds- Lapse of attention/absent mind, Children between 5-12 disappear during puberty.
No preictal--aura or warning, Halo around lights.
No postictal symptoms- very tired.

Tonic-clonic-grand mal-Alternate contraction (tonic) and relaxation (clonic) of the muscle. Whole body jerks
Loss of consciousness- Incontinence during attack.
Preictal-aura
Postictal phase-confused and drowsy.

Status Epilepticus-Rapid continuous seizures, can have absence of breathing. Life Threatening.
Treatment-Treat cause, Epilepsy
Anticonvulsant-Monitor Blood levels
Assessment-Type, Aura, Medications
Help prevent seizure-take meds on time, Factors that trigger a seizure -fatigue, stress, visual, alcohol, caffeine
Interventions-Pad side rails do not restrain,
do not try to pry open mouth for tongue blade-Monitor airway-Assess tongue.
Assess Time began and ended, body parts involved, characteristics of movement, eyes and head deviating, incontinence.
Postictal
Reorient, vital signs, allow to sleep (rest), Patient Education.
Medic alert bracelet participating in activities that could have dangerous effect.

Trigeminal Neuralgia
S & S--severe pain--sharp and intense, 1-2 minute duration; localized on one side of face.
Triggered by exposure to extreme temperature change, chewing, washing face.
Treatment Anticonvulsant– 5th cranial nerve (surgery) nerve goes to ophthalmics mandible and maxilla areas.
Interventions-Nutritional- follow plan, Medications take on time.

Spinal Cord Injury- Classified as :(26 total as sacrum and coccyx is counted as one since there fused)
Cervical-7
Thoracic-12
Lumbosacral-5
Sacrum-5 fused
Coccyx-4 fused
Treatment-Prevent further injury to cord, Repair damage, Establish a routine of care.
Interventions-Immediate care--Always treat as injured until you find out otherwise. Cervical collar, back board, CT to R/O (rule out) injury before removal, log rolling.

Traction-alignment and immobilize =fixate
Crutchfield Tongs = cervical screws in scalp, keeps neck in alignment
try to reduce swelling.
Halo goes around head and shoulders.
Common Problems
1st -Spinal Shock
Bradycardia, hypotension, paralytic ileus
Up to several months-muscles are very flaccid distal to injury.
2nd Muscle Spasms
Initial-flaccid as cord adjusts becomes spastic.
Does not mean return of voluntary function.

Autonomic Dysreflexia-Uninhibited and exaggerated reflex of ANS
to some type of stimuli.
Below Level of Injury -Distended bladder.
Constipation or suppository. Sudden changing of position.
85% of patients at or above T-6
Massive vasoconstriction, seizure, stroke and death.
Above level of injury- Severe pounding headache, elevated B/P,
bradycardia, nasal congestion, profuse sweating and flushing
Below injury-Pallor and goose bumps.

Parkinsonism Degenerative
Disorder, progressive incapacitation -Shaking Palsy-Lack of
Dopamine (neurotransmitter), Idiopathic-not sure what causes it?
S & S Pill rolling--tremors at rest, decrease with voluntary
movement, absent when sleeping and pronounced with stress.
Bradykinesia-poor body balance, difficulty initiating movement;
Gait shuffling, steps short and quicker, absence of arms swinging.
Rigidity-difficulty moving, facial expression becomes mask-like,
speech low and monotone, drooling.
Treatment- Replace dopamine Levodopa=precursor -Sinemet
(levodopa and carbidopa) = keeps in precursor form.
Control tremors, rigidity and drooling-anticholinergics= keeps dried
up / drooling.
Interventions-Preventing complications-Nutrition, soft foods.
Constipation-Increase fluids
Walking, Imagery, Safety-Falls, Tremors and hot liquid.

Multiple Sclerosis

Autoimmune / virus-Affects the CNS--usually progressive. Affects the myelin sheath.

S & S-20-40 years old--Female > male

Motor dysfunction

Sensory dysfunction - eyes

Coordination problems

Mental changes- depression

Fatigue

Unpredictable flare-ups followed by periods of remission.

Diagnosis

Increased IgG Antibody

MRI-white matter lesions

Treatment

Interferon Beta-1 B, Not a cure--reduces attacks by 1/3

Interventions-Supportive measures

Teach-Avoid stress, infections and fatigue-Referral (MS Society).

Alzheimer's

Middle Adult to Older Adult, Slow onset, Progresses at varying rates through several stages-Eventually fatal.

S & S Mental Deterioration

Initial subtle, then progresses, loses ability to think abstractly, exhibit impulsive behavior,

Decline in personal hygiene.

Personality Changes-Usually negative-depressed, suspicious, paranoid, hostile and combative,

Increasing agitation and physical activity.

Speaking skills to nonsense syllables.

Interventions

Calm predictable environment, Reduce anxiety and agitation.

Safe environment

Improve Communications

Promote self-care independence.

Socialization

Adequate Nutrition-one dish at a time.

Myasthenia Gravis
Autoimmune-acetylcholine receptors
Diagnosis
Tensilon-IV given within 1 minute marked increase in muscle strength.
S & S:
Ptosis (drooping eyelid)
Diplopia (double vision)
Dysphonia (impaired voice)
Dysphagia-(difficulty chewing and swallowing)
Treatment
Plasmapheresis-identify what to remove from blood and what to put back in.
Anticholinesterase (Prostigmin) helps with what acetylcholine we have left work better.
Removal of thymus gland.

Interventions
Monitor for excessive Prostigmin dosage.
Poor tongue control, restlessness, anxiety, irritability, difficulty swallowing.
Airway
Nutrition
Fatigue
Weakness
Referral

Head Injury Review
Decerebrate-injury to mid-brain, brain stem-away from chest.
Decorticate-injury to the cerebral cortex-hands to chest.
Posturing-hyperextended neck.
Skull Fracture-severe head injury-toddlers withstand tremendous force before it breaks.
Concussion-temporary confusion or unconsciousness that follows trauma to the brain-jars the brain stem loss of memory before the accident (retrograde amnesia) during & after.
Shaken Baby Syndrome.

Head Injuries
Prevention
Most traumas are preventable! Most victims-risk takers.
Slow down, wear seat belts, do not drink and drive.
Don't drive motorcycles (at least wear helmets)

Predictors of Poor Outcome
Intracranial hematoma
Advanced age
Abnormal motor responses.
Impaired eye movements, absent pupil light reflexes.
Early sustained hypotension, hypoxia, hypercapnia.
IICP more than 20 mmHg

Pathophysiology
HI (HEAD INJURIES) classified in various ways:
1. Amount of actual damage to brain.
2. Whether the brain is exposed (open) or not (closed head injury)
3. Direct injury or indirect contusion, twisting (coup-countercoup, DAI)
4. by three stages of injury.

Stages of HI
Primary HI results directly from injury itself. Does not get any worse.
Skull-, lacerations, abrasions, hematoma.
Secondary **HI**-events that complicate the primary injury, and make the damage worse.
Some preventable. Hypotension, hypoxia,
Hypercapnia, IICP, uncontrolled cerebral edema, infection, malnutrition.

Secondary Injury Mechanism
Ischemia from previous causes disrupts the $Na+ / K+$ ion pump, $Ca+$ channels, capillaries, Become permeable, which reduces lumen size and blood flow is slowed; leukocytes adhere to the walls, of capillaries causing "white thrombi". Biochemical mediators are released, coagulation is stimulated. Neurons become necrotic.

Secondary Injury

Injured areas are hypermetabolic, requiring more 02 and glucose.
HI patient may have other major organ injury, or multi-system failure (lungs, heart, kidney, liver/spleen)
Survival may depend on age, previous health, extent of other injury/shock, immediate care after injury.
Tertiary Head Injury
Results from IICP, which will cause further neuronal ischemia and death.

Skull Fractures

Linear-single line crack. Usually admitted to monitor for brain damage.
Depressed-bone is pressed down into tissue (need surgery to correct)
Comminuted-bone fragmented
Compound/perforated-depressed with scalp laceration. Causes open head injury.
Surgery necessary to clean out blood debris.
Basilar- may cause cranial nerve compression.

Basilar Skull Fracture-Hard to see on x-ray.

Periorbital ecchymosis
(Raccoon eyes) from fracture of frontal fossa.
Mastoid process (temporal bone) ecchymosis (Battle's sign).
From middle fossa fracture. Blood leaks to area of less pressure.

Cerebral Spinal Fluid Leaks

Also from basilar skull fractures.
Rhinorrhea-through nasal passages
Otorrhea-through ear canal (tympanic membrane ruptured)

Tests for CSF:

Spot of blood, with surrounding halo on tissue, after fluid dries.
Positive for glucose
Treatment for CSF Leaks
Keep covered with dry, sterile gauze.
Antibiotics
No blowing nose or coughing. But don't suppress a sneeze.

Coup / Contrecoup Injuries

Usually result from acceleration-deceleration injuries.
Coup is injury to side where impact occurs.
Brain then bounces off skull and hits opposite side-contrecoup.
Causes injury (contusions, tearing) on both sides, can twist brainstem, causing severe injury and death.

Brain Injury Classification

Concussion-Brief, transient reduction in LOC, usually without brain damage, or residual problems.
Watch for up to 48 hrs.
Moderate-Comatose for 20-60 min, with GCS Glasgow coma scale 9-12.
Severe-GCS =Glasgow coma scale less than 8, comatose longer than 1 hr.

Cerebral Contusion

Bruising of brain tissue without puncture of the pia mater.
May occur with cerebral laceration (tearing of cortex).Can occur with blunt or penetrating trauma.
May not cause loss of consciousness. Initial bruise may be small, but secondary injury, (Edema, bleeding) causes major damage.

Clinical Findings-depends on area of injury.
Frontal-hemiparesis, memory loss, judgment.
Temporal-agitated, combative, disoriented, aggressive.
Frontal-temporal-aphasia (Broca's, Wernicke's)
Brain stem-deep coma, decerebrate posturing, death.

Diffuse Axonal Injury

Acceleration- deceleration or rotational injuries (shearing injury, or axonal swelling/ballooning)
Neuronal axons are injured, causing diffuse white matter degeneration and diffuse brain swelling.
(Without focal lesion, infarction, contusion or bleed)
Severe injury can cause death, persistent vegetative state. Most who recover have severe deficits.

Intracerebral Hematoma
Bleeding into the brain parenchyma (tissue) from contusion, laceration, vessel or aneurysm rupture.
Most common in frontal, temporal lobes.
(High mortality rate)
Treatment-craniotomy may be done for trauma. Often can't remove hematoma.

Brain Stem Injury
May be primary injury (contusion) or secondary (edema, IICP, herniation)
-loss of brain stem reflexes, respiratory drive, cardiac function, blood pressure
Management of Brain Stem Injury.
Care of pt with IICP, post craniotomy.
As pt stabilizes, need to prevent long-term complications – pneumonia, contractures, pressure ulcers, constipation.

Complications:
Paralysis, motor weakness, apraxia (inability to perform learned movements, or proper use of object)
Sensory loss or alterations
Visual deficits
Aphasia or communication deficits.
Bowel and bladder dysfunction
Self-care deficits (feeding, hygiene, dressing)
Metabolic and nutritional needs
Disorders of GI function
Cognitive impairment – attention, memory, perception, judgment.
Personality changes, emotional problems, depression, behavioral changes.
Recovery Period, Most recovery in first 6 months.
The sooner there is significant improvement, the better the prognosis.
Steady progress can continue for up to 2 yrs and longer with sustained therapy.
Need ongoing support to accept dysfunctions.

Spinal Cord Injury
Types of Injury
Hyperextension-C4, C5. Greatest amount of damage, greater
backward arc. Soft tissue stretched.
Strained, vertebrae dislocated. Partial dislocation – subluxation.
Spinal cord stretched, contused, ischemic.
Flexion-compresses vertebral bodies, disrupts intervertebral discs.
Usually C5, C6 and lumbar regions.
May cause cord damage. May or may not need surgery.

Hyperflexion-Hyperextension
Usually acceleration-deceleration (rear end or head on collision)
Head thrown forward then rebounds backward.

Whiplash
Soft tissue injury only
Usually rear end collision
Negative x-ray, pain in neck and shoulder, decreased neck movement,
muscle spasms.
May be delayed 12-48 hrs post injury (edema and micro hemorrhages
in muscles and ligaments)
Whiplash Treatment
Non-narcotic analgesics
Local heat or cold
Rest and muscle relaxants
Anti-inflammatory agents
Cervical traction to decrease muscle spasm.

Other Spinal Injuries
Rotation-fractures and dislocations of facets. Several cervical
vertebrae extreme lateral flexion and rotation.
Compression fractures - vertebral body and arch burst and disrupt
ligaments and disc.
Penetration injuries-bullet, sharp object enter vertebral column.

Cervical Cord Injury

C1, C2-rare but often fatal. Immediate loss of respirations.
Fracture unstable, will require surgical fusion, immobilization with halo brace/vest.
Will require permanent ventilator, and caregiver.
Full quadriplegia, little rehab improvement.
C3, C4-Some respiratory muscle function, still need vents.
C5-Partial shoulder and elbow use. Able to hold head up and use a puff-powered motorized wheelchair.
Can use mouth held devices. May be able to feed self with devices.
No bowel or bladder control.
C6-shoulder, elbow and partial wrist use "incomplete or spared quad.
C7-shoulder, elbow, wrist, hand (partial) some degree of arm control,
Certain amount of independence with ADLs with adaptive devices.
May be able to do own rectal stimulation for bowel management.
Can run wheelchair outside, may be able to drive with adaptations.

Care of Cervical Traction

Weights hanging freely
Head down, away from pulley
Clean pin sites according to protocol
Monitor cranial nerves for compression

Turning With Cervical Tongs

Patient rotated from side to side while maintaining cervical traction alignment.
Or log rolling with 3-4 people, keep head and neck aligned.

Halo Traction

Skeletal traction pins attached to metal halo.
Halo attached to hard, form fitting, thoracic vest with metal rods.
Maintains traction, Patient can be more mobile. 2-4 wks after.
Care of Halo Vest
Make sure screws are tight
Have wrench at bedside to open vest for CPR.

Coma

Person is totally unresponsive, unaware of self and surroundings.
Also called depressed level of consciousness.

Pathophysiology

Coma may occur suddenly or gradually as a continuum.
LOC diminishes - takes more intense stimuli to elicit a response.
Thoughts simpler and slower, but more concrete.
Conscious thought is lost, feelings to pain remain. Reflexes become primitive, No response to even painful stimuli, brain death.

Reticular Activating System (RAS) LOC=RAS

Network of nuclei (cell bodies) in brain stem and interbrain (thalamus) that stimulate the cortex, so it can "think". Needed for sleep/wake, concentration, attention, memory and learning.
Disruption of RAS causes coma - interruption of O2, glucose, generalized seizures, trauma, edema, bleeds, increased ICP

Other Causes of Coma

Cortex may become unresponsive to the RAS - cerebral lesions (bilaterally, or compress the other side and brain stem) from edema, neoplasms, blood clots, Alzheimer's.
Metabolic disorders - electrolyte imbalance, hypoglycemia, organ failure, myxedema, Addison's, poisoning, overdose.

Types of Coma
Persistent Vegetative State

Damage in diencephalon or midbrain
Cortical death occurs, but brainstem functions keeping the person alive - respiratory and heart functions continue. Unaware of environment. Usually will not regain awareness after 3-6 months (less than 1 in 100 ever regain self awareness).Aggressive care, then decisions.

Locked-in Syndrome

Not coma, patient aware, alert but paralyzed, unable to respond.
Amyotrophic Lateral Sclerosis (ALS) - still able to blink eyes. Use as communication signal.
* Lou Gehrig's disease.
Communicate professionally.

Irreversible Coma/Brain Death

Complete intracranial circulatory arrest.
Extensive ischemia and necrosis of tissue.
Cortical and brain stem activity ceases, including respirations.
Circulatory failure will occur within 3-5 days (no HR or BP). Organ donation must occur before this.
Diagnosed by clinical exam, supported by EEG, cerebral arteriogram, cerebral blood flow.

Clinical Signs of Brain Death

Deepest grade of coma, no response to pain.
Flaccid muscles (no posturing)
No brain stem reflexes -pupil, oculocephalic (doll's eyes), corneal, ciliospinal (blink),
cough, gag, swallowing, oculovestibular (caloric test).
Pupils-mid-position or dilated and fixed.
No spontaneous respirations (off vent 30 sec)
Second exam (consulting MD) in 12-24 hrs. Spinal reflexes intact - not brain activity

Tests to Confirm Clinical

Most donation protocols require "objective" confirmation.
EEG - "flat line" indicates no brain activity
May not be completely flat, may need to delay donation, risk losing organs.
Cerebral arteriogram - no blood flow definitive.
Portable cerebral artery ultrasound (MCA)
Increased Intracranial Pressure Causes coma and can cause permanent cellular damage and necrosis.
ICP Homeostasis
Skull is rigid, fixed box. Won't expand.
Pressure within cranial vault depends on balance between 3 components:
Brain tissue 80-87 % (tumors, edema).
CSF 9-10 % (500ml produced/24 hrs blockage, decreased absorption).
Intracranial blood 4-10 % (vasoconstriction or vasodilation).

Blood Brain Barrier

Cerebral capillaries-Endothelial cells in vessel lumens and feet of astrocytes create "tight junctions", as well as osmotic and electrical barrier. Result-High degree of control as to types, and amounts of substances that can leave capillary and enter brain interstitial space.

Hemiparesis – one leg everted (turned out, and no fracture exists)

Paralysis - facial droop on one side
Lift both arms and release simultaneously. Paralyzed limb will fall more quickly and flail more.
Test each for resistance to passive stretching.
Response to deep pain.

Cushing's Triad

Hypertension (widened pulse pressure). Can cause neurogenic pulmonary edema.
Bradycardia – CO usually adequate.
Respiratory slowing, pattern depends on pattern of control in area of brain stem still functioning. Will lead to respiratory failure/arrest.
Shock - like VS –medullary CV collapse.

Prevention of Hypercapnia, Hypoxia

Both cause cerebral vasodilation – vessels take up more space and increased ICP. Need endotracheal intubation, mechanical ventilation if GCS < 8. (Sedate with intubation, because CO_2 and ICP increase)
Keep PaO_2 80 – 100 mm Hg
Keep $PaCO_2$ 25 – 30 mm Hg (slight alkalosis to vaso constrict vessels)

Barbiturate Coma

Pentobarbital to induce coma. Used to decrease cerebral metabolic rate and to allow healing to occur.
Brain Attacks Cerebrovascular Accident (CVA) Stroke.
Classification:
Ischemic (no bleed on CT)
– Thrombi
– Emboli

TIAs

Episodes of ischemia lasting 5-30 min, up to 24 hrs.
Symptoms disappear completely when ischemia resolves.
Multiple TIAs with same symptoms-thrombus
Multiple TIAs with different symptoms - emboli
Differences in symptoms depending on whether impairment is from carotid or vertebrobasilar circulation
Both cause hemiparesis or hemiplegia, paresthesia, impairments of vision and speech. Vertebrobasilar – brainstem.
Most common arterial occlusion-middle cerebral artery (MCA). Main stem occlusion wills infarct entire hemisphere.

Thrombolytics

Convert plasminogen to plasmin, which lyses fibrin and releases fibrin degradation products, which inhibit clot formation.
Tissue plasminogen activator (t-PA)
Urokinase (UK), Reteplase, Tenecteplase
Must be started within 3 hrs of symptoms (see ALS guidelines)
Streptokinase – not used in stroke, increased bleeding
Can cause hemorrhage – should be at facility that can deal with head bleed complications.
Avoid inserting Foley within 30 min of t-PA, NG within 24 hrs, if possible.

Chapter 6

Cardiovascular

Acute Coronary Syndrome
New term to describe a range of clinical syndromes representing varying degrees of:
Coronary artery occlusion.
Unstable angina
Non-Q wave MI
Q wave MI
Display chest pain and other symptoms.
Sudden cardiac death can occur with a MI

Hyperlipidemia
Elevated lipids in blood
Cholesterol, triglycerides
Low HDL
High LDL and cholesterol
Saturated fat, calories and refined sugar.

Normal Values
Lipids – 400 – 800 mg/dL
Cholesterol – 120 – 200 mg/dL
Triglycerides vary with age
Men < 40: 46 – 316 mg/dL > 50: 75 – 313 mg/dL
Women < 40: 37 – 174 mg/dL - > 50: 52 – 200 mg/dL

High Density Lipoproteins (good – more protein, carry lipids to liver for metabolism)
Men 44 – 45 mg/dL • Women 55 mg/dL
Low Density Lipoproteins (bad – more cholesterol, high affinity for arterial walls) < 130 mg/dL.
LDL: HDL ratio should be < 3
Controlling levels is key to preventing heart disease.
Elevated levels associated with obesity, inactivity, high alcohol intake, and Tran's fatty acids (fried foods, snack foods)

Common Statins
Statin drugs not only decrease lipids, but they can stabilize, shrink the plaque, decreasing risk of rupture. Also decrease BP, glucose, and mortality.

Atorvastatin (Lipitor)

Fluvastatin (Lescol)

Lovastatin (Mevacor, Altocor)

Pravastatin (Pravachol)

Simvastatin (Zocor)
Most MI's caused by lesions with < 40% arterial occlusion. Soft plaque ruptures with Valsalva pressure.
Larger occlusions (90%) are usually calcified and cause angina.

Atherosclerosis
Arterial intima is injured by LDL, HTN, chemical irritants, bacteria and viruses that cause inflammation. (C-Reactive Protein).
Cholesterol cause thickening of arterial wall.

Endothelial Alteration
Platelets are activated and they release a factor that stimulates smooth muscle growth. The smooth muscle cells entrap lipids.
The lipids calcify and cause an irregular surface, which attracts platelets to adhere and aggregate.

Platelets
When the plaque ruptures the endothelium is exposed to foreign substances. Platelets will adhere and cover the injured site to protect it and allow the healing process to begin.
Collagen in the endothelium activates the platelets to express 70,000 – 100,000 glycoproteins (GP) IIb
IIIa receptors, which release signaling agents ADP, Thromboxane A2, serotonin, and epi.

Platelet Activation
Chemicals released attract more platelets.
Serotonin causes vasoconstriction.
After activation platelets extend pseudopod and express GP IIb-IIIa
receptors that bind with fibrinogen.
This clumps platelets together. They trap RBCs and begin a
thrombus.

Micro embolization
Platelet aggregates are washed downstream and may occlude tiny
arterioles.
Results in ischemia and small infarcts in multiple areas that may only
be detectable by blood tests.
Cause increased risk of CHF and death.

Clot Stabilization
As platelets aggregate, the body produces thrombin. Thrombin
causes unbound fibrinogen circulating around the thrombus to
convert to fibrin.
They form a mesh around the thrombus, stabilizing it and trapping
more RBCs, and macrophages. Thrombus becomes a solid, red clot.

Myocardial Ischemia/Infarction
If unchecked, the clot of RBCs, platelets and fibrin mesh may
completely occlude the coronary artery.
Once myocardial necrosis begins, 500 heart cells die/minute.
The dead cells release Creatine Kinase Myocardial Band, Troponin,
and Myoglobin.

Other Risk Factors
Diabetes - Damages capillary membranes, may affect platelet
aggregation.
Smoking - 20% increase in CO, alters capillary permeability to LDL.
Increases platelet adhesiveness, Aggregation, vasoconstriction.

Angina Pectoris
Not a disease – symptom
Transient inadequate blood flow, unable to meet myocardial oxygen needs.
Ischemia - not permanent muscle loss.

Anginal Chest Pain
May not be described as pain - strangling, aching, tightness, squeezing, pressure, heaviness, dull -not sharp.
Substernal, may be referred to arms (ESP L), jaw, teeth, neck. Watch what patient touches, or rubs. Use the pain scale.
Does it last? 1-5 to 15 min and is it? Precipitated by activity, cold, stress, emotions.

Diagnostic Tests
EKG, enzymes
Exercise or chemical stress test.
Radionuclide imaging.
Echocardiography
Cardiac catheterization with PTCA (percutaneous transluminal coronary angioplasty)
Radionuclide Imaging (Scans)
IV injection of radionuclide to:
Detect "cold spots" from decreased coronary flow.
Evaluate ventricular function
Detect abnormal heart wall motion.
Aneurysm in wall, akinesia (no movement)
Dyskinesia (defective movement)
Done post MI, pre and post.

Types of Radionuclide Tests
Thallium-201 - outlines perfused areas of heart. Used with stress test to evaluate how well heart Perfuses during times of increased O2 demand.
Technetium - localizes necrotic tissue (MI)
Gaited equilibrium heart scan (MUGA) = Multiple Gaited Acquisition, scans synchronized with EKG. Shows wall motion and ejection fraction (normal is more than 55percent)

Echocardiography (ECHO)
Uses ultrasound to outline size, shape, and motion of heart structures (valves)
Non-invasive - large ultrasound probe moved around on chest wall.
Eval patients with chest pain, EKG changes, valve disease, atrial tumors, can now calculate ejection fraction.

TEE ECHO Transesophageal ECHO (TEE)
Ultrasound probe passed down esophagus like a scope. Better visualization through thin tissue, especially posterior wall.

TEE Care
Consent, NPO 6 hrs prior, dentures out.
IV sedation, throat anesthetized with lidocaine spray, bite block.
IV contrast dye may be used.
Post care - frequent vital signs, EKG, and Sp02.
NPO until gag reflex returns.

Electrocardiography
Measures efficiency of heart during stress
1. Exercise - Monitor for chest pain, EKG change on treadmill.
2. Chemical -Meds to ↑ HR, dilate CA = (coronary arteries) using (Persantine, Cardiolite, dobutamine)

Stress Tests
Used to detect EKG abnormalities not normally present at rest.
ST segment changes, rapid atrial or ventricular arrhythmias, heart blocks.
Angina, dyspnea, claudication in legs.
No caffeine, alcohol, smoking 3 hrs before.
Check with Dr Re: heart and BP meds before testing.

Electron Beam Computed Tomography (EBCT)
Non-invasive cardiac CT scan
Three dimensional images of the heart and coronary arteries.
Can reveal coronary artery plaque, calcification, and other abnormalities.

Angiocardiography
Cardiac catheterization.
Percutaneous catheter inserted in femoral artery, aorta, into coronary arteries.
Contrast dye injected to visualize blockages in coronary arteries, detect spasm, and visualize heart motion, valves.
Used in patients with new or worsening chest pain, CHF, abnormal EKG/stress test.

During Cardiac Cath
Dye may cause flushing, warmth, dizziness.
Awake, but sedated.
May be asked to cough - clears contrast from cardiac arteries.

Post Cath Care
Introducer sheath removed (usually in cath lab)
Pressure held above site 10 - 20 min (C clamp or hold pressure manually)
VasoSeal - collagen plug injected in subcutaneous tissue to seal the artery.

Monitoring
Arrhythmias
Hypotension (bleeding, vasodilators)
Acute CA occlusion (MI), stroke or pulmonary embolus from dislodged plaque.
Anaphylaxis or acute renal failure from dye.
Head of bed < 30 degrees, log roll, leg straight 6 hrs (less with VasoSeal), post-op vital signs, leg circulation.
Pressure/sandbag or band-aid

Percutaneous Transluminal Coronary Angioplasty (PTCA)
Balloon catheter used during cardiac cath.
Used to dilate, flatten plaque in occluded coronary arteries.
Can now access multiple, and smaller vessels (flexible)
Less invasive alternative to CABG.

Complications
Coronary artery spasm
Acute artery thrombosis, rupture, MI - need emergency heart surgery team in house.
1/3 to 1/2 develops restenosis in 6 months.

Newer PTCA Techniques
Coronary atherectomy - atherosclerotic plaque is shaved away.
Directional atherectomy - plaque cut by rotating cutter, stored and pulled away. Rotational atherectomy - spinning blades, micro particles of plaque flushed away.
Laser angioplasty - fiberoptic catheter delivers laser to evaporate plaque.

Stents
After artery is opened by angioplasty.
Metal mesh inserted and left in artery.
Incorporated into endothelium.
Help to hold artery open, greatly improving success rates of PTCA (fewer reocclusions).
Requires anticoagulation/anti-platelet meds for at least 1 month.

Treatment of Angina Goals
Provide symptomatic relief (pain, dyspnea)
Prevent myocardial infarction.
Prevent sudden death
Treatment of Angina
Modify risk factors – elevated homocysteine strongest modifiable predictor of morbidity and mortality.
Treat hypertension, hyperlipidemia, DM.
Meds, PTCA/stents

Coronary Artery Bypass Graft surgery (CABG)
Decreasing Homocysteine Levels.
Eat 100 percent RDA of folate (folic acid), and vitamin B 6 and vitamin B 12Vitamin enriched grains and cereals are best. Other foods: vegetables, legumes, meats, fish.

Myocardial Infarction
Ischemic necrosis of portion of muscle.
Produced by interruption of coronary blood flow, from thrombosis or spasm.
Results in permanent loss of contraction in affected myocardium.

Criteria for MI Diagnosis
Must present with 2 out of 3 criteria:
EKG - ST segment or new Q wave.
Characteristic chest pain.
Abnormally elevated cardiac enzymes.

Causes
Same risk factors as angina.
Rapid atrial or ventricular rates, arrhythmias.
Hypotension (hypovolemia)
General anesthesia, stroke.
Endocrine (thyroid) crisis, diabetic coma.
Cocaine

Pathophysiology
Perfusion/oxygenation insufficient.
Cells shift to anaerobic metabolism - produce lactic acid.
Cells die - release chemical mediators (histamine, prostaglandins, kinins, oxygen free radicals). Cause further cell damage.

Types of MIs
R or L ventricle
Subendocardial (non Q wave) - does not extend through whole myocardial wall.
Transmural - involves full thickness of myocardial wall (Q waves develop)

Contributing Factors
Size of infarct depends on: Which artery(s) are blocked (major or distal branch). Collateral circulation - With long standing disease, coronary capillaries **from** another artery may extend to the ischemic area. Will lessen impact of blockage.
Arrhythmias from ischemia can extend damage.

Morphologic Changes

1st 24 hrs - cells edematous, rupture Muscle looks bruised, cyanotic. Leukocytes released.
4-5th days - leukocytes infiltrate, macrophages remove necrotic tissue.
New connective tissue develops, thin (aneurysms in wall can occur)
3 - 6 wks, connective scar tissue.
2 -3 months, scar is well established.

Chest Pain with MI

Severe, crushing, squeezing may be different from angina.
Lasts longer than 15 - 30 min. May radiate wider than anginal pain.
Abdominal pain, heartburn.

Other Signs of MI

Feeling of impending doom, fear, anxiety.
Diaphoresis, cool and clammy (SNS)
Pale, gray, cyanotic, decreased peripheral pulses, blood pressure.
Bradycardia, normal rate or tachycardia.
Nausea, vomiting, diarrhea.
Pulmonary edema - dyspnea, crackles.

Silent MIs

MI may be painless, may just feel ill, or not notice at all.
Atypical chest pain" or no pain - more likely with women, and elderly.

EKG Changes with MI

Zone of necrosis/infarct - tissue dead, no electrical activity of its own. Acts as a window to view activity from opposite wall.
Shows up as Q wave in transmural MI in leads monitoring that part of myocardium.
Zone of injury - area adjacent to infarct. Produces elevated ST segments.
Zone of ischemia - adjacent to injury. Produces T wave inversion, ST depression

Extent of MI
Subendocardial MI
Non - Q wave infarction
Goal: Keep size of infarct as small as possible.
Treatment aimed at decreasing myocardial O2 demand, increasing blood supply
Need to prevent zone of injury and ischemia from converting to infarction.

MI Locations
Anterior - V3, V4
Inferior - II, III, aVF
Posterior - V1 - V4 (reciprocal changes - ST depression) (18 lead EKG on posterior)
Lateral - V5, V6, I and aVL
Septal - V1, V2
R vent - V4R (II, III, aVF)

Cardiac Enzymes and Proteins
Get baseline on admission; follow at regular intervals then daily for several days)

Diagnosing MI
Enzyme and protein elevation only definitive test in all MI patients.
When muscles infarct, enzymes are released by cells, enter circulation.
Some are found only in cardiac muscle.

Traditional Enzyme Markers
Creatine kinase + MB: isoenzyme only found in cardiac muscle (MB)
Rises within 4 - 6 hrs after AMI, peaks in 24 hrs, normal in 3 days.
Sensitive and specific to AMI
Short diagnostic window (can use to detect reinfarction 48 hrs after initial MI)
Can increase with trauma, cardioversion, OHS

CK Normal s
CK < 160 u/L men, < 130 u/L women

New Protein Markers
Cardiac Troponin, Myoglobin
Troponin complex plays a role in contraction of cardiac muscle.
3 proteins: cardiac troponin T, I, C.
Amino acids in T, I different in cardiac vs. skeletal muscle.
Troponin/Myoglobin
Small molecular size
So leak out of cells soon after injury.
T and I not found in blood of healthy adults.
Presence indicates myocardial tissue death.
Cardiac Troponin **T**
Sensitive and specific indicator of AMI.
Normal < 0.1 ng/mL
Elevates in 3 -5 hrs, remain up 14 - 21 days.
Also released in unstable angina.
Decreased ↓ Specificity for AMI, useful for ischemia.
Can also be released with acute muscle disease,
Trauma, chronic renal failure (false +)

Cardiac Troponin I
Sensitive of AMI within 6 hrs
0.5 – 2.0 ng/mL nonspecific myocardial injury.
> 2. Ng/mL myocardial injury.
Very specific, only found in cardiac cells.
Not affected by cardioversion, OHS, renal.
More useful than CK-MB (affected by surgery, cardioversion).

Prognosis
Stronger prognostic value in unstable angina (>0.4 predicted
increased mortality)
Prolonged elevation - may mask increases from reinfarction.

Myoglobin
Heme protein found in skeletal and cardiac muscle. Smaller than CK-MB molecules.
Can detect 2 hrs after AMI (60 percent within 3 hrs, 100 percent within 6 hrs).

Can't use to definitively rule in MI - affected by: skeletal muscle, neuromuscular disorders, strenuous exercise, IM injections, CABG, ETOH.
But - if it's normal within the lst 3 -6 hrs, AMI can be ruled out.
Normal range 50 -120 mcg/ml.
Use as earliest indicator, with combination with other markers.

Ischemic Chest Pain
Initial Assessment
Vital signs, IV access
12 lead EKG
Brief, targeted history and exam, Cardiac enzyme levels, Portable chest x-ray

Morphine
Primarily dilates veins, reducing preload.
Mild arterial dilation that reduces afterload.
Decreases SNS overload from pain (decreases HR, vasoconstriction)
Lowers BP, so need to monitor closely.

Oxygen
Reduces myocardial workload
Hypoxemia can lead to cardiac arrhythmias and organ failure.

IV Fluids
MI patients can become dehydrated.

Thrombolytic Agents-Infusions which dissolve thrombi.
Best success occurs within the 1st hour symptoms begin.
After 6 to 12 hrs, no statistical benefit.
Try to begin within 1st 6 hrs.
Tissue plasminogen activator (t-PA).
Streptokinase
Urokinase
Anisoylated plasminogen activator complex (APSAC)
Retavase (newer, faster/better results)
Tenecteplase (TNKase)
Alteplase (Activase)

Complications-Bleeding from thrombolytic or anticoagulant drugs. Monitor for hypovolemia, respiratory changes-dyspnea, and tachypnea.
Neurological changes-LOC-Loss of consciousness, restlessness.
Skin-hematomas, bleeding puncture sites.
Hematuria (red or brown), hematemesis, melano (black)

Anticoagulant Therapy-Instituted with thrombolytics to lessen further thrombus development.
Aspirin 325 mg chewed, crushed, SL when chest pain begins. ASA within 1st 24 hrs reduces mortality.
Heparin drip
Integrilin-inhibits platelet aggregation.
ReoPro-platelet receptor GP llb/llla, inhibits aggregation.

Other Medications-Beta blockers **significantly** decrease mortality by decreasing cardiac oxygen demand,
Response to catecholamines (decreased HR), and controlling arrhythmias,
Inhibiting renin production (decreased BP and Na+ and H2O retention).
Nitroglycerine IV drips-venous dilation, decrease preload, dilates coronary arteries.
ACE inhibitors-decrease BP, NA+ and H20 retention.

Other Interventions-Foley cath to monitor hourly urine output – 0.5 ml/kg/hr (30 cc minimum in adult)
Anti-anxiety agents for sedation to decrease SNS, increase rest.
Diet-clear liquids to reg AHA, low Na and fat, no caffeine.
Stool softener, use commode instead of bedpan.

Psychological Considerations-Angina and MI are very frightening events.
Patients need calmness, confidence and teaching along the way.
Very scary to transfer out of ICU. Need to address fear as normal.

Intra Aortic Balloon Pump (IABP/IACP)

Catheter with inflatable balloon is threaded through the femoral artery into the descending aorta.

It is inflated with helium or CO2 by a machine that is attached to an arterial line.

The balloon is timed with the patient's cardiac cycle, so that it inflates during diastole, and deflates during systole.

IABP Effect-During diastole, the inflated balloon pushes blood up into the coronary arteries to improve perfusion.

As systole is occurring, the balloon deflates quickly, causing a pressure gradient. The blood rushes out of the LV to fill the void, thus decreasing afterload.

Allows the heart to rest and heal.

Complications of IABP

Very invasive and potentially dangerous.

Bleeding, infection, loss of perfusion to leg, gas embolism.

If timing is off, can greatly increase afterload (heart pumping against inflated balloon)

Need advanced training, and 1:1 with the pump to change timing with HR changes.

Weaning IABP

Monitor for improved BP, CO and U/O

Wean off or decrease inotropic drips.

Decrease the balloon support from 1:1 to 1:2 then 1:3

Balloon removed by Dr.

Left Ventricular Assist Device (LVAD)

Pulmonary vein cannulated, oxygenated blood pulled from heart and pumped back into the aorta.

Rests the ventricle

Coronary Artery Bypass Grafts (CABG)

Veins or arteries are sewn into the coronary artery, above the blockage. They bypass the blockage, and are sewn in distal to it, providing blood flow to the muscle.

Techniques

Patient is placed on cardiopulmonary bypass (extracorporeal circulation) to oxygenate and pump the blood.
Blood anti-coagulated, warmed.
Heart is cooled and stopped (cardioplegia) with iced saline and KCL
Grafts are sewn, heart warmed, defibrillated, bypass removed.

Bypass Grafts

Venous – usually saphenous vein from medial leg, direction reversed in heart to keep vein's valves open.
Arterial – internal mammary. Most common graft.
Still connected to arterial supply, one end is grafted onto coronary artery. Can remain patent longer than veins.
Radial artery grafts now being used.

Complications

Ischemic myocardial injury/AMI, Arrhythmias
Limb ischemia-monitor peripheral pulses closely for thrombo emboli.
Hemorrhage-Monitor mediastinal chest tube drainage (normal < 100 ml/hr)
Hypovolemia-patients warm up post-op, vasodilate. Fluids monitor.
Electrolyte imbalance-low K+, Ca+, Mg+
Respiratory complications- on vent, sedate wean and extubate night of surgery.
Infection-sternum, vein donor site (leg)
Post - op fever-inflammatory response.
Gastric distension-NG post-op, D/C next day.
Neurological ischemia-emboli, hypotension.
Post Pump Psychosis-agitation, hallucinations from anesthesia, sensory overload, sleep deprivation.

Newer Techniques

Minimally Invasive Direct CABG (MID CABG)
Thoracotomy incision used, heart bypassed while still beating. Avoids splitting sternum and cardiopulmonary bypass. Limited candidate use.
Transmyocardial Revascularization
Small hole (1 mm) burned into the ventricle

Hemostasis on outside of heart achieved by direct finger pressure. Blood from ventricle enters the small channels to perfuse the tissue (based on reptilian circulation)

Cardiac Reduction Surgery
Scarred, dysfunctional portions of heart muscle are removed. Allows remaining healthy muscle to contract more normally, to improve cardiac output.

Chapter 7

Respiratory

Chronic Obstructive Pulmonary Disease
COPD
Chronic bronchitis - History of excessive secretion of bronchial mucus and productive cough for >3 months, two years in row.
Smoking - only identifiable cause
Emphysema - Permanent, abnormal enlarged air spaces distal to terminal bronchioles. Destruction of alveolar walls.

Epidemiology
Smoking. Smokers develop COPD, but it's the principle cause of death in 80 - 90% of those with COPD.
May link with genetic factors to cause disease.

Risk Factors
Highest risk - cigarette smokers. Next - pipe and cigar
Improvement of symptoms and pulmonary function does occur after quitting.
Genetic Factors - Deficiency of alpha1-protease inhibitor.
Naturally occurring proteolytic enzyme.
May inhibit substances that initiate the emphysema process.

Occupational/Environmental
-Chronic exposure to chemical fumes, dust (silica, cotton), and exhaust fumes.
-Still less risk than smoking
-Causes allergies and respiratory infections.
-Predisposes to COPD (especially if coupled with smoking, and genetic factors)

Affective State
-Depression and anxiety common

Nursing Management

Nurse counseling to stop smoking increases compliance.
Refer to local "smoke stoppers" programs.
Set a good example - stop smoking yourself!
Refer to genetic counseling (for alph1 antitrypsin deficiency)
Wear masks - dust, cold, polluted air.
Prevention teach to :(avoid crowds, get pneumonia and flu vaccines)

Chronic Bronchitis

Pathophysiology
1. Bronchial irritation and inflammation
2. Hypertrophy of mucous glands
3. Hypersecretion of mucus
4. Impaired mucociliary clearance
5. Bronchospasm
Stagnant mucus is medium for viruses and bacteria, increases mucus.
Coughing - progressive injury to bronchioles.
Bronchial walls ulcerated.
Loss of ciliated epithelium.
Scarring-stenosis, fibrosis.
Destroys small bronchioles, narrows larger. Alveoli
Obstruction/inflammation
Decreased Ventilation and diffusion
Decreased PaO_2 and increased $PaCO_2$

Pulmonary Vasculature

Hypoxia causes reflexive pulmonary artery vasoconstriction.
Increased PAP (pulmonary artery pressure)
Pulmonary hypertension (R vent afterload)
R side heart failure - cor pulmonale.

Result

Frequent infections
Inflammation, Edema
Increased mucus
Large and small airway fibrosis.
Emphysema

Pathophysiology
Two main types-Centrilobular, Panlobular.

Centrilobular
Begins at center of pulmonary lobule and extends outward toward periphery.
Causes impaired gas exchange.
Associated with smoking, chronic bronchitis.

Panlobular
Uniform destruction of all alveoli distal to terminal bronchioles with progressive loss of tissue
Problem - decreased alveolar-capillary surface area (V: Q mismatch)

Both Types
Inflammation, infection, retained secretions and mucosal congestion.
Causes bronchiolar obstruction.
Loss of elasticity, increased airway resistance.
Repeated inflammation - stimulates overreaction of macrophages.
Causes alveolar tissue digestion.

Alveoli
Large, dilated, serum filled
Emphysematous blebs - up to 1 cm diameter.
Emphysematous bullae - > 1 cm diameter.
Wall elastic recoil decreased - airways collapse.
Increased resistance, slowing of airflow on expiration.

Ventilation
Damage not uniform, some areas better than others.
Increased $PaCO_2$ (hypercapnia) - respiratory acidosis, causes increased RR.
Medulla desensitized to increased $PaCO_2$
Hypoxic drive develops - brain now depends on decreased PaO_2 (hypoxia) to stimulate respirations.

Bronchitis
Frequent, productive cough.
Bronchospasm, frequent respiratory infections.
DOE, dyspnea on exertion, History of cigarette smoking.
Hypoxemia and hypercapnia – hypoventilation from airway resistance.
Polycythemia (Hgb 20 gms), cyanosis (at least 5 gms Hgb unsaturated) - blue bloater.
Normal to overweight frequently develops centrilobular emphysema

Emphysema
Dyspnea, DOE
Minimal coughing, no sputum.
Air trapping, flattened diaphragm, barrel chest.
Hypoxemia may be present (with exercise)
Hypercapnia late in disease. Pink puffer.
Thin, hypermetabolic state working to breathe. Protein malnutrition.

Diagnostic Studies
Chest x-ray
Sputum analysis
Pulmonary Function Studies:
-Forced Vital Capacity (FVC) - maximum expiration after maximum inspiration
-Forced Expiratory Volume in 1 sec (FEV1) - amount of air exhaled in 1 second

FEV1-forced expiratory volume in one second
 Correlates with prognosis.
 Less than 80% of expected value - airflow obstruction.
Abnormal FEV1 - administer bronchodilator and retest in 30 min.
Asthma patients - improvement in FEV1.
Bronchitis patients - may improve.
Emphysema pts - no change in FEV1.

Lung Capacities
Established bronchitis- decreased FEV1 and increased residual volume
Emphysema - Total lung capacity increased, but there's decreased air available for respiration (vital capacity decreased), because residual volume increased.

ABG's
Chronic Bronchitis - severe hypoxia and hypercapnia.
Respiratory acidosis - kidneys retain bicarb to try to buffer/compensate pH.
Emphysema-At first, some hypoxia and minimal hypercapnia-compensated by hyperventilating.
Respiratory acidosis occurs later in disease.

CBC
Increased RBCs to compensate for hypoxemia.
Increased Hgb/Hct
(Hgb> 20)
Polycythemia

Treatment
 First needs to quit smoking and live in a smoke free environment.
Alleviate acute symptoms/prevent complications
Low flow O2
Bronchodilators
Antibiotics
Corticosteroids
Adequate fluid intake

Oxygen Therapy
2 -3 l/min with PaO2 less than 55mmHg or polycythemia.
R ventricular hypertrophy, signs of cor pulmonale:
(Hepatomegaly, JVD-jugular vein distention, peripheral edema)
Goal 65 -80 mmHg or sat 88 - 90 %
Use at least 15-18 hours every day.

Bronchodilator Inhalers

Anticholinergic (anti vagal)-Ipratropium bromide (Atrovent),
Tiotropium bromide.
(Spiriva HandiHaler -breaks capsule, inhale powder)
Even more effective than B2 bronchodilators in emphysema.
Combivent (ipratropium and albuterol)

Bronchodilators

Beta2 adrenergic agonists
Theophylline is a weaker bronchodilator
Improve respiratory muscle function and mucociliary function.
Aminophylline, Theo-dur
Watch for/ teach signs of toxicity.

Other Medications

Broad Spectrum Antibiotics - bacterial infections (purulent sputum)
Mucokinetic agents - liquefy mucus.
Lung Reduction Surgery

External High Frequency Ventilation (EHFV)

Uses mask/nose clip
Assists with ventilation
Uses small tidal volumes (1-5 ml/kg) and rapid rates (100 – 300
breaths/min)
Allows respiratory muscles to rest
Decreases $PaCO_2$ and increases PaO_2 and O_2 sat

Corticosteroids

Controversial with COPD
May use as trial if large number of eosinophils (increase in allergies)
in sputum and obstruction that can't be decreased with
bronchodilation. Try for 1 wk, continue if improvement occurs. May
use every other day.
Inhalers - avoid systemic complications (GI bleed, osteoporosis,
cataracts, and psych.

Complications
Bronchopulmonary infection
R side heart failure (cor pulmonale)
Acute respiratory failure
Ventilator - may take weeks to wean, become vent dependent.
Duodenal ulcers and GERD - stress, vent, nicotine, steroids and B2 drugs.

Prognosis
Nursing Management.
Goals - maintain patent airways.
Facilitate O2 and CO2 exchange.
How? - improve pulmonary hygiene.
-Avoid irritants (smoking)
-Adequate hydration
-Cough, postural drainage, Flutter device.
-Meds - bronchodilators, antibiotics.

Nursing Management
Relieve bronchospasm.
Increase exercise tolerance gradually.
Pulmonary rehab
Treat concurrent infections.

Psychosocial Needs
May see great personality changes dealing with chronic disease.
Anger/guilt (from smoking?)
Fear of death
Fear of not dying - living debilitated as pulmonary invalid.
May require full time caregiver, role change.

Fatigue
Always present
Always SOB, no break.
Sleep disrupted no control of respiratory in REM. So avoids REM, sleep cycle disrupted. Wake suddenly with SOB.
Sex - too SOB-shortness of breath, need info, and support.

Nutrition
Proper nourishment essential
Will break down respiratory muscles for energy (catabolism)
High risk for malnutrition:
Bronchodilators - gastric irritants.
Sputum may alter desire/taste of food.
Dyspnea - interferes with prep and eating.

Nutrition Indicators
Weight
Serum albumin and transferrin.
Total iron-binding capacity.
Creatinine
Zinc

Diet Guidelines
Carbohydrates (CHO) produce more CO_2 than protein and fat when metabolized.
Need diet higher in protein, fat, calories.
Lower in CHO
Avoid foods causing gas/bloating.
Simplify meal prep, rest before eating.
Eat in quiet, relaxing atmosphere.
Eat multiple small meals.

Nursing Care Plan
Teaching coughing techniques.
Pursed lip and diaphragmatic breathing.
Hydration
O2, meds, and rest

Chapter 8

Reproduction

Reproduction Review

Gamatogenesis-tracing heritage from both mother and father.

Chorion-fetal membrane closest to the posterior uterine wall and gives rise to the placenta.

Decidua-uterus lining called endometrium where the maternal side of the placenta arises.

Germ Layer-The germ layers of the embryo are the exoderm, mesoderm, and endoderm. All structures of the individuals develop from these layers.

Amniotic-the Chorion and the Amnion together form the bag of waters.

Age of viability- at twenty weeks gestation the lungs have developed enough to survive outside the uterus.

Wharton's Jelly-covers and cushions the cord vessels to keep them separated (two arteries carry blood away from the fetus and one vein returns the blood)

Dizygotic-Fraternal twins two separate fertilized eggs.

Monozygotic- Identical twins same egg.

Male & Female Reproductive Systems

Puberty:

Male-penis, grows hair

Effects of Testosterone-increase muscle mass, strength, long bones, enhance RBC, penis, descending teste.

Growth Changes between 13 16. Years

Female breast development, before menses.

Effects of Estrogen & Progesterone-broad hips, breasts, hair, menstrual cycle.

Ovum-

Life cycle

Terminology

Spermatozoa-male germ cell, reproduction of spermatogenesis.
Ovum-female germ cell.
Ovarian follicle-cavity that contains a single ova.
Oogenesis-formation of germ of ova.
Corpus luteum-empty follicle after ovulation.

Female A & P

Uterus

Endometrium-implantation, hormone changes, sloughs off every month with menses, 30-60cc loss menses.
Myometrium-expel baby.
Perimetrium-keep shape of uterus is a serous layer and has some muscle.
Cervix-lubrication of the vagina walls, bacteriostatic, alkaline.
Fallopian Tube-outer 3rd site for fertilization, route for ova.
Ovaries-below and behind fallopian tube, estrogen, progesterone.
Breast-4 lobes, warm shower, suckling also causes milk to come in.
Pelvic Function-all part of birthing process.
Supporting and protecting pelvic contents.
Forms a relatively fixed passage for baby.
Support and distribute body weight.
Most important muscle-levator ani.
To support the urethra, vagina and rectum.

Bones of the Pelvis

Two innominate bones; each consists of a/an
-Ilium
-Pubis
-Ischium
-Sacrum 5 and Coccyx 4- tailbone

Pelvic Deviations

True pelvis-below ischial spine True pelvis – consists of the inlet, pelvic cavity and outlet.

-Linea terminalis

False Pelvis above the pelvic brim.

-Supports the enlarging uterus and guides the fetus into the true pelvis.

Female-born with 1 million ova, 400,000 by puberty, over lifetime only 400 ova fertilize.

Young moms have a lot of downs syndrome. A sperm life 24-72 hours is alkaline.

Pelvic Measurements-distant between the ischial spine, transverse most important 13cm/5.25in.

Pelvic Inlet Anteroposterior, Transverse, Right left oblique.

Pelvic Cavity-Has many, most important is the interspinous, Caldwell-Moloy Pelvic

Gynecoid- normal best for delivery.

Android-male posterior outlet reduced, usually have C/S.

Anthropoid- A shape, 25% has this deliver posterior.

Platypelloid flat, posterior anterior, baby cant progress down.

The Ovarian & Endometrial Cycle knows when estrogen is high and low.

Menstrual phase Days 1 through 5 of cycle.

Estrogen & progesterone levels decrease.

Elevate FSH & steady levels of LH.

Stimulate ovulation and development of the corpus luteum.

Initiates estrogen secretion by the ovary.

Proliferative Phase (follicular) Days 6 through 14.

Increased Estrogen Production

Proliferation of Endometrium and Myometrium in preparation for implantation.

Follicle secretes estradiol.

FSH production decreases before ovulation.

Approximately day 14

(Luteal) Secretory Phase Days 15 to16.
Corpus Luteum formed under the influence of LH.
Estrogen and Progesterone production increased.
Endometrium is prepared for implantation of fertilized ovum.
Ischemic Phase Days 27 to 28.
Corpus luteum degenerates if conception does not occur.
Estrogen and Progesterone levels decline if conception does not occur.

Common Terms

Conception-sperm enter the ova.
Zygote-fertilized ovum.
Mitosis-division of cells.
Implantation-zygote implanted.
Decidua-endometrium after implantation.
Chorion-closest to uterus.
Amnion-onion skin layer.
Embryonic Disc -placenta-raise for development of fetus, layers of embryo develop here.
Lunar Month- 28 days
Yolk sac 1st 6 wks, provide RBC production, base of core as fetus grows it disappears.
Blastocyte- gives 3 prime layers-wherever this implants the placenta grows.

Fertilization Prenatal Development Three Stages of Prenatal Development.

-Zygote-Fertilized Ovum.
-Embryo-2-8th week development-oogenesis
-Fetus-9 weeks to birth- fetus is growing development.
-Placenta-1.5 lbs, life of placenta 41 wks.
-Organ for fetal respiration, nutrition, and excretion.

Produces four hormones

-Progesterone maintains lining; prevent abortion, location, teste on male fetus.
-Estrogen blood flow, lactation, uterine growth.

-Human chorionic gonadotropin (hCG) - pregnancy test causes corpus luteum to persist.
-Human placental lactogen (hPL) decreases insulin sensitive – increases glucose.
Cord-AVA-2 arteries 1 vein, 50-55 cm, 2 cm around, blood travels 400ml/minute. Mom lay of left side best for fetal circulation.

Fetal Circulation

Changes in circulation after birth.
Maternal-Fetal Circulation
Development of the Embryonic Disc-3 germ layers, anionic fluid is produced by mom, baby urine.
Amniotic fluid –insulates warms, facilitates growth, cushions fetus, collects waste
Ectoderm- nerve, epithelium, lenses.
Mesoderm-smooth muscle, ct, BVS, teeth, pleura lining of eye, pituitary, kidney, ureter.
Endoderm-respiratory and GI, lining of the GI.
Heart beat 6 wks-110-160 bpm-longer gestation heart rate gets slower.
FHT Doppler-10 weeks, 37-40 weeks normal gestation
Lightening-baby drops
Fetoscope-1/2 way through the pregnancy.
Test LS ratio- lecith ion and sphingomyelin, tells fetus can live outside utero.

Abortion-Miscarriage

Abortion - any intentional or unintentional demise of the fetus or evacuation of the uterus.
Legal/moral/spiritual consider.
Spontaneous (non-intentional)
-Threatened-vaginal bleeding occurs.
-Inevitable-membrane ruptures, cervical dilation.
-Complete-everything evacuates including placenta.
-Incomplete-needs D/C.
-Missed-fetal death <20 weeks usually need D/C.
-Recurrent-more than 2-3 missed abortions.

-Induced–therapeutic (abortion abnormalities & elective (personal choice)
Full term 38-40 weeks.
Preterm 28 -37 weeks- 33 weeks will have possible respiratory problems.
Extreme preterm- to 27 weeks.
Very Extremely preterm-23 to 25 wks- 23 wks 500g-(1.1lbs) viable to live outside uterus with help.

Abnormal Gestations
Abortion -any intentional or unintentional demise of the fetus and evacuation of the uterus. Legal/moral/spiritual.
Pre-maturity -birth prior to 37 weeks.
Post-maturity -birth at 41 weeks- baby gets stressed, longer overdue heart rate drops.
Viability -ability of the fetus to survive outside the uterus.

Function of Genes-male determines sex, xy male, xx female.
Chromosomes, Sperm, Ovum, Human Cell, Sex determination.

The Process of Fertilization and Implantation
When does fertilization occur-sperm and ova.
Where does fertilization occur-upper 1/3 of fallopian tube.
Where does implantation occur-blastocyte implants in the endometriosis of the uterus-which gives rise to placenta.

Twins
Identical-one of everything except for 2 amnions placenta is shared, monozygotic, same sex, same egg splits.
Fraternal-have two of everything dizygotic-2 eggs and has its own placenta, chorion and amnion.

Autosomes-22 pair of Autosomes and 1 pair of sex chromosomes.
Teratogen-causes damage to growing cells in the womb.
Diploid-a body cell of 46 chromosomes.
Spermatogenesis-process of mitosis in the sperm.
Oogenesis-process of mitosis in the ovum.

Haploid-having 23 unpaired chromosomes.

Fertilization-when the sperm and ova unite when fertilized there are, -23 chromosomes from the sperm and 23 from the ova returning to the diploid number of 46.

Gamatogenesis- tracing heritage from both mother and father.

Chorion- fetal membrane closest to the posterior uterine wall and gives rise to the placenta

Decidua- uterus lining called endometrium where the maternal side of the placenta arises.

Germ Layer- The germ layers of the embryo are the exoderm, mesoderm, and endoderm. All structures of the individuals develop from these layers.

Amniotic- the Chorion and the Amnion together form the bag of waters

Age of viability- at twenty weeks gestation the lungs have developed enough to survive outside the uterus.

Wharton's Jelly- covers and cushions the cord vessels to keep them separated (two arteries carry blood away from the fetus and one vein returns the blood)

Dizygotic- Fraternal twin's two separate fertilized eggs.

Monozygotic- Identical twins same egg.

The uniqueness of each individual result from the blending of genes on the 46 chromosomes contained in each body cell and the environment of the embryo and fetus during development.

-Gamatogenesis in the male is spermatogenesis. Each mature sperm has 22 Autosomes, plus either an X or Y sex chromosome for a total of 23. Gamatogenesis in the female is called Oogenesis. It begins at ovulation and is not completed until fertilization occurs. The mature ovum has 22 Autosomes plus the X sex chromosome for a total of 23. At conception the total number of chromosomes is restored to 46.

-When the ovum is fertilized by X sperm female results a Y sperm will be male.

-After fertilization in the fallopian tube the zygote enters the uterus where implantation is complete by seven days after fertilization. If the zygote fails to move through the tube implantation occurs there and a tubal entopic pregnancy occurs.

-When implantation occurs in the uterine lining the cells of the zygote differentiate and develop into the following structures, Chorion, amnion, yolk sac, and primary germ layer. The Chorion develops into the embryonic/fetal portion of the placenta, the amnion encloses the embryo and amniotic fluid, the primary germ layers develop into different parts of the growing fetus, the yolk sac which functions only during embryonic life, begins to form red blood cells.

-The germ layers of the embryo are the exoderm, mesoderm, and endoderm. All structures of the individuals develop from these layers.

-All body systems are formed and functioning in a simple way at the end of the eighth week.

-The accessory structures of pregnancy are the placenta, umbilical cord, and fetal circulation. These structures continually support the fetus throughout prenatal life in preparation for birth.

-The placenta is an organ for fetal respiration, nutrition, and excretion. Is a temporary endocrine gland that produces progesterone, estrogen, human chorionic gonadotropin (hCG), and human placental lactogen (hPL).

-Fetal circulation transports oxygen and nutrients to the fetus and disposes of CO2 and other waste products from the fetus. The temporary fetal circulatory structures are the foramen ovale, ductus arteriosus, and ductus venosus. They divert most blood from the fetal liver and lungs because these organs do not fully function during prenatal life.

Bi-ischial diameter-the distance between the inner surfaces of the ischial tuberosities.

Climacteric-any ova that remaining at (time surrounding menopause)

Diagonal Conjugates-the distance between the suprapubic angle and the sacral promontory.

Obstetric Conjugate-inlet diameter estimated by subtracting 1 ½ to 2 cm from diagonal conjugate.

Transverse Diameter-the largest diameter of the inlet and determines the inlet shape.

Four types of pelvises: Gynecoid, Anthropoid, Android, Platypelloid.

Dyspareunia- pelvic weakness or painful intercourse.

Embryo-fertilized ovum (egg)

Internal Os-the opening near the uterine corpus.
External Os-the opening near the vagina.
Fetus-developing structure from the 8th till birth.
Menarche-the first menstrual period.
Menopause-final menstrual period menopause and climacteric are often used interchangeably.
Ovulation-discharging a mature ovum from the ovaries 14 days before menses.
Ovum-egg
Puberty-secondary sexual characteristics develop.
Rugae-transverse ridges of the vagina.
Semen-seminal plasma and sperm together that is called semen.
Smegma-cheese like secretion of the sebaceous glands.
Spermatogenesis-mature spermatozoa are formed and number of chromosomes are reduced by half.
Zygote-a fertilized ovum.

-Testosterone is the principle male hormone. Estrogen and Progesterone are the principle female hormones. Testosterone secretion continues throughout a man's life, but estrogen and progesterone secretions are very low after a woman reaches the climacteric.
-The penis and scrotum are the principle male genitalia. The scrotum keeps the testes cooler than the rest of the body promoting normal sperm production.
-The two main functions of the testes are to manufacture sperm and secret male hormones (Androgens, primarily testosterone).
-The myometrium (middle muscular layer) is functional in pregnancy and labor. The endometrium (inner layer) is functional in menstruation and implantation of a fertilized ovum.
-The female breasts are composed of fatty and fibrous tissue and glands that secret milk. The size does not influence the ability to secrete milk.
-The female reproductive cycle consists of regular changes of hormone secretions from the anterior pituitary gland and ovaries, maturation and release of an ovum, and builds up and breaks down of the uterine lining.

-The glenoid pelvis is most favorable for vaginal birth.

-The pelvis is divided into a false pelvis above the linea terminalis and the true pelvis is below this line. The true pelvis is most important in birth and is further divided into the pelvic inlet, cavity, and outlet.

The Birthing Process

Lightening-drop 2 weeks before labor in first pregnancy- leg cramps.

Braxton Hicks contractions-false labor- usually in front groin area.

Cervical changes-ripen, soft, spongy, because of prostaglandins we produce.

Bloody show-24-48 hours of labor, progesterone makes this mucus membrane.

Rupture of membranes-12-24 hours, strep, pulmonary hypertension for baby.

Gastrointestinal disturbance-indigestion, heartburn, diarrhea, nausea, vomiting is common.

Sudden burst of energy- 2 days prior to labor- nesting.

Maternal Systemic Responses to Labor

Cardiovascular system- increased cardiac output when have contraction, no blood available to baby.

Respiratory- Continuous O2

Renal- down in true pelvis blocks bladder, cath patient.

Gastrointestinal-decreased Peristalsis

Fluid Electrolyte balance-increased temperature and increased sweating.

Imune system-base CBC, stress on body increased WBC always when body is stresses.

Integumentary-perineum- warm oil midwives put on. Doctor cuts this area.

Neurological- endorphins increase, pain threshold sensitive effect.

Components of the Birth Process

The four P's of the birth process.

-Powers-uterine contractions, maternal pushing.

-Passage-bony pelvis, soft tissue.

-Passenger-Fetus, fetal head.

-Psyche-expectations of birthing process.

Mom has no idea how much pain involved so explain about pain meds that are available.

The Powers:
Uterine Contractions
Primary power of labor during 1st stage.
-From onset till complete dilation of cervix- important to know.
-Effacement - thinning of cervix - % - needs 100%
-Dilation-opening of cervix-cm-10.
Phases of Contractions:
-Increment-period of increasing strength.
-Peak-period of greatest strength.
-Decrement-period of decreasing strength.

Contractions
Frequency-beginning of one to beginning to another 2 minutes.
Duration-beginning to end or length of one contraction.
Intensity-strength
Interval-times uterus relaxed between contractions- less than 90 minutes fetus is in trouble.
Differentiation between True & False Labor.

TRUE contractions get shorter never longer.
-Regular Contractions –frequency is the same.
-Discomfort begins in the back and spreads to the abdomen.
-Progressive cervical dilation & effacement.
-Intervals between contractions gradually shorten.
-Intensity of contractions increases with ambulation.
-Contractions increase in duration & intensity.

FALSE
-Irregular Contractions
-Discomfort localized in abdomen.
-No change in cervical dilation & effacement.
-No change in or irregular contractions.
-Ambulating has no effect on contractions
-No change in duration or intensity of contractions.

Maternal Pushing
-When fully dilate-voluntary pushing to assist with contractions.
-Propels fetus downward through the pelvis.
-Premature urge to push before fully dilated because fetus pressing on rectum.
-Exhaustion, epidural may reduce desire to push.
The Passage:
Bony Pelvis
-False Pelvis
-True Pelvis
Inlet at top
Mid pelvis
Outlet near the perineum
Soft Tissue
Up -5
-4
-3   FAKE – ischium spine up
-2
-1
-0
+1
+2
+3   TRUE – ischium spine down
+4
+5

The Passenger:
The Fetus and The Placenta- molding usually parietal bone goes back to normal.
Fetal Head
-Anterior fontanel ◊ frontal, parietal bones join (coronal suture) sideways.
-Posterior fontanel- Δ sagittal- lamboid bones/sutures 2 parietal and occipital bones.
-Fetal Lie Longitudinal Lie – up and down- how baby is aligned to mom's spine.
-Transverse Lie- across.
-Oblique Lie- sideways.

Attitude-normally one of flexion.
Presentation - fetal part enters pelvis first.
-Cephalic (head first) head down.
Vertex - head fully flexed- best for delivery.
Military - neither flexed not extended.
Brow - partially extended- in opening in cervix
Face - head is fully extended- in opening of cervix- face first delivered.

Breech Presentations

-Frank Breech - legs extended toward the shoulder.
-Complete Breech - butt first with flexion of head and extremities.
-Footling Breech - one foot dangling.
-Double Footling Breech - both feet dangling.
-Shoulder presentation- lying transverse shoulder is presentation.
Position - how a reference point on the presenting part is oriented to the mother's pelvis.
Occiput - head in cephalic
Sacrum - breech presentation

Pelvis - 4 sections
-R & L anterior (front quadrant)
-R & L Posterior (back quadrant)
Understanding Abbreviations
First Letter - R or L side of pelvis
-May be omitted if directly A/P
Second Letter - Fetal preference point
Occiput –vertex
Mentum-face
Sacrum-breech
Third Letter - Anterior/posterior/Transverse
Bregma (brow/face) - may be used

The Psyche:-therapeutic is good to find out what beliefs they hold.

Mental state
-Relaxed/optimistic
-Mark anxiety/increase pain/decrease tolerance.
Catecholamines - inhibit uterine contractions.
Cultural influence, Does not dictate behavior
People are individuals within their culture.

Mechanisms of Labor
Engagement-fetal head reaches ischial spine.
Descent- moving down thru pelvis.
Flexion- head moves to chest.
Internal Rotation-enters pelvis occiput is R or L; contractions make head turn directly under pubis occiput.
Extension- head must change form flexion to extension to make the curve.
External Rotation- doc usually- shoulders are crosswise in pelvis.

Admission of a Client in Labor:
Labor is Different for each person.
Priorities include establishing a nurse/client relationship.
Assessing the condition of mother and fetus may be undertaken in a sequential order.

Nursing Process Assessment:
Subjective data: comfort of mother, her ability to cope, need to urinate, defecate.
Objective data: vital signs; FHR; frequency, duration, interval, and intensity of contractions; fetopelvic relationships; condition of membranes; maternal behavior; maternal verbalizations.

Nursing Diagnosis:
Impaired verbal communication.
Pain, Fatigue, Anxiety, Fear, Deficient knowledge, Risk for infection.
Risk for deficient fluid volume
Impaired urinary elimination, Impaired (fetal) gas exchange
Altered tissue perfusion (maternal)

Impaired physical mobility
Ineffective coping
Risk for injury

Planning the Outcome Identification
Client:
Shows progress through labor.
Expresses satisfaction with assistance.
Maintains adequate hydration.
Voids at least every 2 hours.
Actively participates in labor process.
Does not experience any injury.

Nursing Interventions:
Assessment, timing contractions, and listening to FHR regularly.
Comfort measures
Hygiene measures
Ambulation and position
Food and fluid intake
Elimination
Breathing Techniques:
Provide adequate oxygenation of mother and fetus.
Provide a focus of attention.
Decrease pain and anxiety.
Increase mental and physical relaxation.

Pharmacologic Comfort:
Systemic medications, Epidural block, Intrathecal block, Local
infiltration, Pudendal block, General anesthesia.
Induction-Augmentation of Labor:
Induction—stimulation of uterine contractions before they begin
spontaneously. Pitocin and monitor.
Augmentation—stimulation of contractions after spontaneously
beginning, but with unsatisfactory progress.
Induction via amniotomy: artificial rupture of membranes.
Induction of Labor best transport baby inside mom.
Readiness for Induction

-Fetal maturity- LS ratio- amniocentesis measures surfactant in baby lungs.
-Cervical readiness
-Fetal position

Risks of Labor and Birth:
Preterm labor and birth <37 weeks
Premature rupture of membranes
Dystocia- shoulder is stuck. Do c/s or break baby clavicle.
Abnormal duration of labor not over 24 hours.
Prolapsed cord- hidden occult
Cephalopelvic Disproportion (CPD)
Precipitate Labor
Fetal Distress

Cesarean Birth:
Birth of an infant through an incision in the abdomen and uterus.
Scheduled or unscheduled.
Pediatrician is usually present to care for the infant.
Some clients may be able to have a vaginal birth with next pregnancy.
Forceps-Assisted Birth:
Forceps are metal instruments used on fetal head to assist in delivery.
Cervix must be completely dilated and membranes must be ruptured.
Position and station of fetal head must be known.
Newborn possible facial bruising, edema.

Vacuum- Assisted Birth:
Indications are same as for forceps-assisted birth.
Maternal risks include vaginal and rectal lacerations.
Fetal risks: cephalhematoma, brachial plexus palsy, retinal and intracranial hemorrhage, hyperbilirubinemia.

Maternal Evaluation- go to hosp. contractions are regular 5 minutes apart for an hour.
Para 10 minutes apart for hour.
During Labor
Manifestations of Progress. -Dilation- how cervix is opening.

-Effacement-is it thinning and moving up.
-Station-relationship to head and ischial spine.
-Elimination
-Hydration
-Contractions

Fetal Heart Rate monitoring 110-160- below 100 crash c section.
Early deceleration of FHR- caused by head compression, HR comes
down a bit before contractions.
Late deceleration of FHR- big problems- not enough O2, placenta
O2 deficiency. Reposition mom sometimes will help. Variable
deceleration of FHR- umbilical cord compression V, W, U on strip.
Accelerations of FHR15 beats a minute over baseline during
contraction is good.
Variability of FHR
Increased Variability of FHR
Decreased Variability of FHR

Fetal Assessment
Fetal Blood Sampling
ph of baby's scalp- at 2 cm at station 2 to check for blood gasses.
Good 725or above/ 720 or below crash =c/s. = severe hypoxia
-Definition
-Procedure
-Conditions
-Results
External & Internal Monitoring – external Doppler transducer /
toco transducer after 1-2 cm dilated.
Coaches Role during Labor.
Provide emotional support.
Provide physical support.
Enhancing communication.
Reducing anxiety and pain perception.
Aiding in the initiation of bonding.

First Stage: Dilation and Effacement-4 phases of labor the 1st phase has 3.

Begins with onset of regular contractions and ends with cervical dilatation.

The longest stage of labor. Divided into three phases: latent, active, and transition.

Latent Phase: Ends when cervix is dilated 4 cm.
Contractions become more frequent.
The duration of contractions becomes longer.
Intensity of contractions becomes more moderate.
Mother is usually alert and talkative.

Active Phase: pain meds at this stage. Begins when cervix is dilated 4 cm, ends when the cervix is dilated 8 cm.
Contractions occur every 3 to 5 minutes with duration of 40 to 60 seconds.
Intensity progresses to strong.
The client focuses more on breathing techniques in contractions, less talkative.

Transition Phase:
Begins when cervix is dilated 8 cm, ends when cervix is dilated 10 cm. Contractions occur every 2 to 3 minutes with duration of 60 to 90 seconds.
The intensity of contractions is strong.
The client needs to be reminded to focus, relax, and breathe with each contraction.

Characteristics of the Transition Phase:
Restlessness
Hyperventilation- fast breathing. Diaphoretic/ paper bag will help here.
Bewilderment and anger., Difficulty following directions.
Focus on self- getting baby out and how much it hurts.
Irritability

Nausea, vomiting- emesis basin, is common in this phase.
Very warm feeling
Perspiration
Increasing rectal pressure- baby head on rectum.

Second Phase Birth of The Baby-1-3 minutes contraction
"crowning."
Begins when cervical dilatation is complete and ends with birth of the
baby. .
Now that cervix is completely dilated, the mother can actively push.
An episiotomy (an incision in the perineum) may be performed.
Midline is the most common/anus. Medial lateral L-R diagonal cut.

Third Stage Delivery of the Placenta 2-3 lbs
Begins with birth of baby and ends with delivery of placenta.
Should occur within 30 minutes or less.
Birthing facility disposes of the placenta after delivery.
Occasionally, client asks to have placenta to uphold cultural
expectations.

Fourth Stage Recovery immediate postpartum #1 priority is
hemorrhage.
First 4 hours after the birth.
Blood loss is usually between 250 mL and 500 mL.
Uterus should remain contracted to control bleeding, positioned in
the midline of the abdomen, level with the umbilicus.
Mother may experience shaking chills. Warm blankets for comfort.
Schulte fetal/smooth.   Duncan maternal/rough.
If uterus deviates R mom has full bladder.

Care of the Infant:
A–airway- bulb syringe
B–breathing
C–circulation
W–warmth- being cool-being cool increases respirations.

Apgar Score- 10 is best done once then at 5 minutes.
2- Heart rate>100
2-Repirations- good crying
2-Muscle Tone- Active Motions
2 Reflex Irritate- cough, sneeze, cry
2- color- complete Pink

Care of the Mother:

Take blood pressure before and after administration of oxytocic medication.
Fundus of uterus should be firm, size of grapefruit, in midline, below umbilicus.
Episiotomy is washed and dried.
Maternity vaginal pads are applied.
Mother and infant are allowed to bond.

Lacerations-1-4 degrees

Vaginal mucosa and skin of perineum.
Vaginal perineum and levator muscle.
Entire perineum and external sphincter of anus.
Entire perineum sphincter of anus and wall of uterus.

Incisions:

Vertical incision likely never to have a vaginal birth again.
Transverse incision can have vaginal birth.

Postpartum:

Puerperium- the six weeks following childbirth referred to as the fourth trimester of pregnancy.
Involution- changes that the reproductive organs particularly the uterus undergo after birth to return to pre pregnancy size.
Uterine lining- called endometrium when not pregnant and decidua during pregnancy.
After pains- intermittent uterine contractions similar to menstrual cramps decreases 48 hours postpartum.
Lochia- vaginal discharge after delivery composed of endometrial tissue, blood, and lymph there are three stages.
Rubra-blood three days after birth.

Serosa pink-blood and mucus three to ten days after birth Alba clear or white ten to twenty-one days after birth.
One gram of weight equals one milliliter of blood.
REEDA
R=Redness
E=Edema
E=Ecchymosis
D=Discharge
A=Approximation (intactness of the suture line.
Post Partum blues-joy and emotional letdown the first few weeks after birth.
Colostrum-late in pregnancy first few days after birth,
-this is secreted rich in protective antibodies vitamins A and E and essential minerals.
Traditional Milk-The first 7 to 10 days has fewer immunoglobulins but an increase in lactose fat and calories.
Mature Milk-14 days after birth bluish in color has 20 kilocals an ounce and all the nutrition an infant needs.
Suckling-Giving or taking nourishment at the breast. 0.14ml to suck and 0.01ml per suck.
Infant nurses 10 to 15 minutes per breast 8 to 10 times a day.
Homan's Sign-Pain on the dorsal flexion of the foot.
Patient experiences pain in the calf of the leg an indication of thrombophlebitis.

Important Points to Remember
-It is essential to consider each patient individually to better incorporate their special needs into their plan of care.
-From its level at the umbilicus the uterus should descend about one fingers width per day it should no longer be palpable ten days post partum.
-A slow pulse is common in the early post partum period. A maternal pulse rate that would be high normal at other times may indicate hemorrhage or post partum infection.
-A full bladder interferes with uterine contractions which can lead to hemorrhage.
-Measures to prevent constipation should be empathized at each assessment, fluid intake, a high fiber diet, and activity.

-RhoGAM is given within 72 hours to the rh-negative mother who delivers an rh positive infant.

-A post partum check should include the status of fundus, lochia, breast, perineum, bowel and bladder elimination, vital signs, Homan's sign, pain and evidence of parent infant attachment.

-Neo natal screening tests such as the Phenylketonuria (PKU) identify disorders that can be treated to reduce or prevent disability.

-Nurse must always keep the possibility of infant abduction in mind when providing care.

-Bonding and attachment require contact between parents and infant, the nurse must promote this contact whenever possible.

-More breast milk removed equals more milk produced.

-Duration of nursing on the first breast should be at least ten minutes to stimulate more milk production.

-A nursing mother needs 500 extra calories a day plus ten glasses of water.

-Weaning from the breast should be gradual.

-Three major formula types are Modified Cow's Milk Soy Protein or Protein Hydrolysate

.-Diastasis Recti longitudinal abdominal muscle that extends from the chest to the pubis symphysis is separated during C-section

-Galactagogue breast milk stimulators brewer's yeast, rice, gruel, fenugreek tea, and sesame tea used post partum.

Post Delivery Care of Mother and Baby
Handwashing is #1 for OB and PEDS
Epidural-monitor B/P, Hypertension
Intrathecal-Itching, use Benadryl
Post-partum period
-Puerperium
Fundus -Involution- return uterus to non productive state.
-After pains- contraction of uterine, release from Pit, Oxytocin, also breast feeding.
-Lochia-Vaginal discharge- not menstruation.
-Atony- Boggy fundus - needs massage to tighten back up.
-Engorgement- hard, vascular and lymph feeding in for milk, warm compresses.

The Fourth Stage of Labor (Immediate Postpartum Period)
Time Frame
1-4 hours after delivery of the placenta - normal gushing while massages.
Nursing Responsibilities
-Identifying and preventing hemorrhage.
-Evaluating and intervening for pain.
-Observing bladder function and urinary output -6 hours if not voided cath-check for latex allergies.
-Evaluating recovery from anesthesia lay flat for 6 hours- check for feelings to return
-Promoting bonding and attachment
Nursing Assessment-Postpartum

BUBBLE-HE
-B-Breast -2-3 days PP, full/soft milk comes in wear firm bra.
-U-Uterus-5-6 weeks back to normal, 6-7 weeks placental site healed afterpains 48 hours.
-B-Bladder- displaces uterus to RIGHT if full. Cath, I&O, 1-3 voids minimum (15oml).
-B-Bowel-bowel sounds, frequency of bowel \movement, color, consistency.
-L-Lochia- huge shift in blood volume. Red 3 days, pink/mucus3-10 days, white/alba 10-14 days. Scant1", Light4" Moderate 6"
Heavy>6" or 1 pad saturated every 2 hours, Excessive every 15 minutes.
-E-Episiotomy -Ice every 48 hours REEDA.
-H-Homan's Sign- pain in café, dorsiflexion, indicates possible thrombophlebitis or Thrombus (Measure Cafe).
-E-Emotional state.
Average bloodloss-500ml for delivery and 1000ml for Cesarian section.

Breast

2 - 3 days PP full & soft
3rd day PP firm & lumpy (milk production begins)
Engorgement (nursing & non-nursing)
Hard, erect, very uncomfortable
Nursing assessment
Check for consistency, size, and shape if a lot of dimpling follow up with doctor.
Nipples: redness, cracking- buff with towel.
Flat, or inverted
Supportive garment
Use of breast pumps & shield

Milk:

Yellow Colostrum- immune globulins for 3 months
Blue Hue, Transition
Watery Blue – sweet 4-5 days
Foremilk-thinnest
Hind milk-last fat

Rubin's' Phases-Take in/self, Take hold/Teach Let go/Reality.
PPB-post partum blues 1-72 hours.
PPD-post partum depression 3 days to 6 weeks after.
BUFFA- baby up for adoption.

Uterus

Return to pre pregnant state week's 5-6-involution.
Placental site completely healed by 6-7 weeks.
Firm-grapefruit
Ascend within hours of delivery than descends.
After pains-48 hours

Uterine Assessment-Measure the top of the fundus in finger breaths above, below or at the umbilicus.
If massage is necessary. "Uterus: boggy to increase firmness with light massage".
Sometimes Pitocin will help with this if massage doesn't work.

Bladder
Displaces uterus when full
Higher than expected
Deviated to one side usually right
May feel soft

Empty bladder
Amount (min. 150 ml)
1st 2-3 voids
Frequency
Assisting client

Bowel
Assess bowel sounds (c- section)
Frequency of bowel movements. Color & consistency.
Measures to prevent constipation
Drink adequate fluids. Add fiber to diet.
Ambulation a must
Hemorrhoids- from pushing

Episiotomy- assess Mom laying on her side- use flashlight
Redness /pain
Edema at or around site
Ecchymosis-bruising or hematomas
Discharge-from the site
Color, odor, amount
Approximation-well approximated
Sutures intact
Nursing Interventions ice packs-1st 48 hours, cleaning, tucks/witch hazel and pain meds.

Lochia
Lochia rubra
Red, composed mostly of blood
Last-3 days PP
Lochia serosa
Pinkish-composed of blood & mucus
Last-3-10 days PP

Lochia Alba
Whitish, mostly mucus
Last-10-14 days PP
Amount of lochia in 1 hour
Scant Less than 1 inch (2.5 cm) stain.
Light-small   Less than 4 inch (10 cm) stain.
Moderate-Less than 6 inch (15 cm) stain.
Large or Heavy Greater than a 6 inch (15 cm) stain or saturation of pad in 2 hours.
Excessive-Saturation of pad in 15 minutes.

Homan's Sign

Pain in the calf with dorsiflexion of the foot.
Indicates thrombophlebitis or thrombosis-watch for red/swelling/heat.
Controversial
Emotional State
Assess for weepiness
Depression
Family support
Interaction with family members.

Postpartum Care

Perineal care should be done after each void & Bowel Movement.
-Sitz bath
Remove perineal pad from front to back.
-Avoid contamination of urinary meatus or vagina.
Average blood loss 500 ml for NSVD and
-1000 ml for Cesarean births
Vital Signs
-Report Temp > 100.4F (esp. after 1st 24hrs)
-Monitor Blood pressures closely.
-Monitor Pulse & RR per hospital protocol.
Return of Ovulation
Six to Eight Weeks – for return of normal menstrual cycle.
Nursing mothers 2 to 18 months.
-May not have a menstrual cycle but can continue to ovulate.

Lactation
Hormonal influences during pregnancy.
Begin 1ˢᵗ trimester
Ductal sprouting (estrogen)
Ductal branching (estrogen)
Lobular formation (progesterone)
Prolactin (manufactures breast milk) rapidly produced after placenta removed.
Oxytocin-(post-pit)
Alveoli-milk producing sacs
Duct system
Nipple-milk ejection/let down.

Stages of Human Milk
Colostrum
Transitional milk
Mature milk
Fore Milk
Hind Milk
Nutritional Needs
Additional 500 calories daily. Follow a well balanced diet using the Food Pyramid.
Avoid caffeine, gas forming veg., chocolate & strawberries.
Medications-check with health care.

Maternal Immune System
Rh immune globulin (RhoGAM).
-Give to prevent sensitization of Rh negative mothers with Rh positive erythrocytes from an Rh positive fetus.
-Give at 28 weeks and within 72 hours of delivery.
-Intramuscular injection-deltoid.
-Rubella immunization
-Should not become pregnant within three months.
-Do not give if allergic to Neomycin or had a blood transfusion within 3 months.
-Common Side effects: rash, slight fever, malaise, sore throat, headache, joint pain.

Attachment - Bonding

Rubin's Three Postpartum Psychologic Phases.
-Taking In-passive & willing to let other do for her-has great interest in infant but others can provide care.
-Taking Hold-Interested in care, critical of performance, ideal time for teaching.
-Letting Go-Give up fantasy child so they can accept the real child.
Parent contact that enhance bonding.
Touching baby, looking at the baby, and holding the baby.

Postpartum Blues vs. Depression

PPB-an emotional effect of childbirth,
Consisting mainly of transient feelings of sadness for a period of about 72 hours.
-Weepiness, mood instability, anxiety, confusion about feelings.
-PPD – an abnormal psychiatric condition occurs 3 days to 6 weeks after childbirth.
-Mild PPB to intense suicidal depressive psychosis.
-1/3 of PP mom's experience to some degree.
-No preparation for childbirth, unrealistic plans for PP work/travel, denies responsibilities of parenthood.
-BUFA- baby up for adoption.

Caring for the Grieving Family

Therapeutic Communication
-Express grief
-Accept & Encourage expressions of feelings.
Support Cultural Practices of Family
Prepare family for what infant will look like.
-Cloth infant
-Expose most "normal" appearing parts.
Memory Packets
Grief Symbol on door/cardex/medical record.
Review Independently
Cultural Influences on postpartum
Postpartum Care Plans
Changes in the body systems

Immediately After Delivery
Dry
ID baby
Assess-Apgar scores 0-2 due to hypoxia low blood sugar, respiratory, low O2.
<5 do another in 10 minutes.
Life threatening conditions
RDS, Apnea, HR, Seizures
Vital Signs
-Umbilical cord/cord blood
-Weight/Length/Head (around brow) & Chest circum. (around nipples)
-Gestational Age Assessment

Newborn Characteristics
6-9 pounds
2700 gms to 4000gms
19 – 21½ inches
46-56 cms
HC 13.2 to 14.8 inches
33.5 to 37.6 cms
HR 110 to 160 BPM
RR 30 – 60
A -Temp 97 – 100 F if <97 document/ intervention.
36.1 – 37.8 C

Normal Characteristics & Deviations
Acrocyanosis-blue hands /feet.
Epstein's Pearls- in mouth-normal from vernix.
Lanugo- body hair
Milia-white bumps on face, vernix in cells and is normal do not squeeze.
Molding-head occipital and parietal bones cross over.
Mongolian spots-dark skin, sacral/wrists/ankles look like bruises will go away by 2.

Cephalohematoma-does not cross suture line/hard/blood filled.
Caput Succedaneum-cross suture lines /Edema.
Fontanels
Erythremia Toxicum-rash looks like flea bites.
Hypospadias-meatus on bottom side (dorsal of penis).
Epispadias-meatus are on top (dorsal) of penis.
Icterus Neonatorum-Jaundice, high Bilirubin, yellowing of skin.
Telangiectatic Nevi-stork bites /red marks.

Reflexes

-Moro- startle reflex/ clap hands, baby will expand arms and legs then back to normal position.
-Rooting/Sucking touch baby will turn head 1st 6 weeks of then they can see the nipple.
-Babinski-toes fan out, heal at J shape. Lasts 5 months.
-Tonic Neck-on back extends body parts the side their looking and the other side will flex.
Palmer grasps reflex-6 -3 months baby grab your finger.
Planter grasp- 8-9 month's press on ball of foot toes will curl down.
Stepping reflex- up to 4 months like their walking as u hold them, then they push up on their own.

The Newborn at Risk & Appearances

Preterm < 37 weeks-Term 38 – 40 weeks-Post Term - > 40 weeks.
SGA-below 10% regardless of gestation.
LGA-wt above 90th %
IUGR-Growth retarded
AGA-Appropriate for gestational age.
Perinatal Factors that place infant at risk
Maternal health history-mom who has heath problems.
Complications of Pregnancy or Labor-PIH, gestational diabetes.
Size & Gestation Age
Difficulty of Birth- dystocia or prolapse cord or o2.
Narcotic administration within 1-1½ hours of birth.
Precipitous-fast delivery.

Thermoregulation

Evaporation- parents bathing infant slowly

Conduction- infant placed on cool padded surface for assessment-transfer of heat to cooler area.

Convection-Air-conditioning vent blowing air on infant-loss of heat to surrounding area.

Radiation – Infant's crib located near window on a cold day.

Brown Fat Location-at term- kidneys, back neck and scapula -lose 10% of this fat right away.

97.7-98.6 axillary / 99.6 rectal.

Methods to Reduce Hypothermia

Drying-reduces evaporation heat lost.

Hat-reduces heat loss through the head-Head is 25% of skin surface-Apply to dry head do not use under warmer.

Radiant Warmer-adds supplemental heat.

Parent contact-Skin to skin warming- Kangaroo care, body to body to keep warm.

Umbilical Cord

Umbilical cord-finger breath above umbilicus.

Three vessels- 2 Arteries-carries blood away from baby- 1Large.Vein-carries blood and nutrients to baby.

Vessels supported by Wharton's Jelly- keeps from kinks.

Normal length-12 to 36 inches or (30 to 90 cm).

Vitamin K- Aqua- MEPHYTON

Newborns have temporary Deficiency in Vitamin. K

For formation of clotting factors manufactured by bacteria in the intestines. Needs to eat to form bacteria.

Intestinal tract is Sterile every birth until normal flora is established, must have food to produce bacteria.

Always given intramuscular in the anterior thigh 0.5 to 1 mg 5lb or less 0.5mg (Vastus Lateralis)

Ophthalmia Neonatorum-purulent conjunctivitis & keratitis of newborn eyes from exposure to gonorrhea and chlamydia.
Public health department requires all infants be treated with.
Erythromycin ophthalmic ointment following birth- leave in 1 minute, signs of infection must be cultured.
Fontanelle- allows brain to grow.
Anterior-Diamond Shape 2 parietal bones & 2 frontal bones Closes at 12 to 18 months.
Posterior-Triangular in Shape 2 parietal bones & one occipital bone closes by end of 2nd month.
Function: allow head to adapt to diameter of the birth canal & allow for future growth.
Craniostenosis- fontanelle closed- surgery to open to allow brain to grow.

Vital Signs
Apnea: >15 seconds: not uncommon: count for one full minute.
Heart Rate-2 types of murmurs frequently heard.
-Functional: is normal and due to blood passing through the normal heart valves.
-Organic: due to abnormal openings or normal openings that have not closed yet.
Temperature: Initial is usually rectal then axillary.

Musculoskeletal Assessment
Movements are random & uncoordinated.
Eyes often appear cross-eyed –nystagmus normal.
Tremors during crying are normal. Constant tremors during sleep may not be normal.
Muscle tone – should not be limp- would be signs of cardiac or hyperglycemia.

Newborn's Kidney Function
Blood flow - ⅓ of adult renal blood flow.
Reabsorption functions:
-Short renal tubules limit capacity to reabsorb substances.

Glucose, amino acids, phosphates, bicarbonate- insufficient surfactant.
-Limited ability to concentrate urine.
-Limited ability to cope with fluid imbalances.
-Fontanelle s sink in if dehydrated- should be flat also mucus membranes will be dry and skin turgor.

Circumcision
Yellen or Gomco-Plastibell- never use Vaseline on this one, bell is put on and tied skin necrosis and falls off.
Pros-Prevention of premature CA, Fewer UTI's-Decrease in transmission of STD's.
Cons-Hemorrhage & infection.
AAP- (American academy of pediatrics) do not support circumcision- Cosmetic and Strictly parental choice.

Newborn Stools
Meconium: green- black, thick & sticky passed 8 – 24 hours after birth.
Transitional: loose & green-yellow, contain mucus usually gone 1st week.
Breastfed infants stool: yellow soft & pasty may have 3 to 6 per day or every time they feed.
Bottle fed: yellow-brown, more solid and fewer in numbers.
Abnormal stools:
-Small putty-like-liver problems.
-Diarrhea
-Bloody stool- possible fissure if bright red is on outside of stool, do cultures to be sure for fetal or maternal blood.

Feeding Infants- 120 cal per kg per day
Forms of Formula: ready to feed single use, ready to feed cans, concentrated liquid, powder.
Never prop a bottle
Do not heat in microwave
Discard leftover formula- most 4 hours.
Position on back or side
Newborn Screening

PKU-mandatory in every state- build up of PKU- control by diet, causes retardation- most blonde blue eyed.
Hypothyroidism-cause growth failure- can take Synthroid rest of life.
Galactosemia-intolerance of lactose (milk sugar) - special diet.
Sickle cell disease- transfusion- interferes with carry of O2.
Thalassemia-polypeptide chain deficiency of alpha and beta production.
Maple Syrup Urine Disease- metabolism- amino acids-urine smells sweet
+ 32 other test.

Physiologic Jaundice
Normal occurrence
Excess RBCs are destroyed after birth because baby breaths air & get oxygen directly.
The high Hct (large number of erythrocytes) is unnecessary after birth.
Appears 2 to 3 days after birth last about 7 days- direct sun works great if in range.
Treatment: Based on levels bilirubin <25, phototherapy, mask only, blanket therapy don't need goggles.

Discharge Instructions
Rest
Hygiene
Sexual intercourse
Exercise
Diet
Nine danger signals that the PP mom needs to report immediately.

Postpartum Complications-Hemorrhage
4th stage of labor 2-4 hrs after delivery of placenta.
Blood loss >500 cc VD- and <1000 cc CS-may include amniotic fluid.
Early Post partum occurs within 24 hours of birth.
Causes-uterine atony-(boggy fundus) or retained placenta.
Nurse: Uterine massage until firm (avoid over stimulation) - teach patient how to do this and Empty bladder.

Late PP treatment after 24 hours up to 6 weeks.
Pain- breast feeding releases oxytocin helps with contractions, contraction increase the more kids you have.
Changes in lochia- rubra 3d, serosa 3-10d, Alba 10-14days- sex is not suggested before bleeding stops.
Vital Signs-temperature stays up with infection.
Fundal assessment

BUBBLE HE-breast, uterus, bladder, bowels, episiotomy-Homans sign, emotions.
REEDA-redness edema, ecchymosis, drainage, approximation.

Hypovolemic Shock
Anxiety (early) confusion, restlessness & lethargy.
Pale, cool and clammy.
Increased Heart Rate, Increased Respiratory Rate is early signs.
Blood pressure changes.
Pulse pressure narrows initially example.120/80=40.
Decreases as shock progresses
Eventually undetectable

Infections
Temp of 100.4 >24 hours after birth -Occurring on the 2nd day of the 1st 10 days.
-Localized signs-redness, edema & pain.
-Systemic symptoms-fever, malaise, ache & loss of appetite.

Nutritional demands change
Need food high in protein (meat) & Vitamin C (citrus, green leaf vegetables) to promote healing.
Increase Iron intake to correct anemia- because of big fluid shift.
Education on aseptic technique-wash front to back.
Treatment-antibiotics- if breast feeding be sure it's ok.
UTI-encourage fluid intake of 3liters/day.
Foods to increase urine acidity-Apricots, cranberry juice, plums & prunes normal PH 5.0-8.

Mastitis (in milk ducts)-Inflammation of the breast generally during breast feeding 2-4 weeks after birth.
Usual cause-Staphylococcus aureus-Maybe Candida albicans.
Factors-Crack or fissure in Nipple- Breast engorgement.
Soreness-shorter feeding time allows for milk stasis (inadequate emptying).
Nurse: Antibiotics-and Heat application Heat: Increases blood flow to the area- Promotes comfort- Promotes emptying.

Subinvolution of the uterus

Delayed return of the uterus to a non pregnant state- (usually takes 6 wks)._Characteristics-Fundal Height greater than amount of time since birth.._Persistence of lochia rubra or slowed progression through the phases of lochia.

Reproductive System and Stressors

Female-Diagnostic Tests
-BSE-know the norms for that patient, breast self exams has not decreased mortality of the disease.
-Pelvic Exam/Pap -scrape cervic cells, start as soon as menses start, has decreases morbidity.
-Colposcopy/Laparoscopy-visual for abnormalities, can biopsy, which is #1 way to diagnose cancer.
-D & C-for missed abortion or miscarriage.
-Mammography
-Sonogram- uterus or ovary
Nursing Process- Assessment- menses, how long, hard, flow, regular, mood, cramps, sex activity, and multiple partners.
Discharge, burn urination, contraceptives, how many kids, any STD's, last pap smear and mammogram.

Nursing Diagnosis- Altered Body Image.

Menstruation
Amenorrhea-without
Dysmenorrhea-painful
Metrorrhagia-bleed between menses.

Menorrhagia-assistive amount at menses.
Stressors
Breast Cancer- Surgery
PID- pelvic inflammatory disease.
Sexually Active- Risk Factors- multiple partners and IUD's.
S & S- None to pain, fever, foul smelling discharge.

Endometriosis- Endometrial tissue outside of uterus.
S & S-pain and adhesions
Treatment
Hormone therapy-birth control.
D & C-helps for a short time.
Hysterectomy

Fibrocystic Breast Disease-Reproductive year's hormone shift.
S & S-lumps in breast- tender before menses- because of hormone shift unilateral and bilateral.
Caffeine and salt aggravates menses.

Breast Cancer- cancer cells floats in lymph nodes.
Family history-females on mother's side- menopause start around 50.
Early onset of menses/late menopause- genetics.
Nulliparity (NO) or the 1st child was late.
FBC- fibrotic breasts.
High-fat diet
Diagnostic Tests- Mammograms/BSE
S & S Lump in breast-usually tenderness.
Retracting and/or abnormal discharge from nipple.
Dimpling
Swelling, increased firmness.
Redness, dry flaky areas
Treatment
Lumpectomy
Partial mastectomy
Total mastectomy
Modified radical
Radical- takes all of it. Reconstructive after mastectomy.

Preoperative
-Education, bras, implants
Postoperative
-Monitor bleeding/pressure dressing, mastectomy, circle spot on dressing, and look under body for blood.
-B/P and IV's unaffected arm
-Exercises- front wall, side wall climbing, rope around door for circular motion, stick lift above head.
-Reach to Recovery- talk with people, who had the surgery, they want to see the incision sign of acceptance.

Male Reproductive
Causes- Inflammation/infection
History of undescended testicle
Genetics
STD's
Hygiene

Prevention
Sexual Partners /Condoms
Good hygiene
Testicular self-exam
Yearly PSA and Digital Exam and check for occult blood.

Diagnostic Tests
Digital Rectal
Testicular Self-exam-lumps, masses, palpate groin because of lymph nodes.
PSA-prostate specific antigen, routine lab increased levels.
Transrectal Ultrasonography of Prostate.
Biopsy- cells

Nursing Process
Assessment- urine change, sex, premature ejaculation, lumps, masses, drug alcohol use, hypertension, vasectomy.
Palpate groin area, transillumination for blood flow and masses.
Nursing Diagnoses
Urinary retention

Anxiety
Pain
Sexual Dysfunction
Body Image Disturbance

Epididymitis-Caused from, STD's or vigorous exercise.
S & S- groin pain, scrotal pain and swelling.
Treatment
Bedrest, ice packs, scrotal support and elevation.
Antibiotics (STD's treat partner)
Avoid lifting, straining and sex.

Benign Prostatic Hypertrophy (BPH)-Hesitancy, dribbling,
difficulty in starting, decreased stream of urine.
Post-operative care TURP- transurethral resection prostrate, most
common, tape cath to leg, no drainage means a clot block.
Drink lots of water 12-14 glasses.
Teach no lifting, sports or sex, cath care, fever, cloudy urine.
Proscar (androgen)-suppresses Testosterone.
CBI -continuous bladder irrigation- holds 1000cc drain in and back
out, increase or decrease flow by urine color.
Dribbling for up to 6 months.

Sexually Transmitted Diseases (STD's)
Nursing Process
Assessment-what age sex, partners, drug use, pain, discharge, look for
soars, discharge, odor, color.
Nursing Diagnoses
-Knowledge deficit
-Pain
-Anxiety/Fear

Chlamydia
Males-dysuria, frequency, discharge- blisters on glans penis.
Females-asymptomatic, discharge, itching- found on pap smears.
Diagnosis-gram stain
Treatment for partners
Venereal Warts-HPV-highly contagious.

Cauliflower-like growths.
Diagnose-Biopsy, pap, Colposcopy
Treat-freezing, laser-no known cure.

Genital Herpes- Herpes Simplex 1-oral and 2 vaginal.
Highly contagious pus filled vesicles even before breakout.
Painful intercourse
Vesicles, burning genital pain.
No known cure.
Increase fluids, ice packs, Sitz bath, clean and dry.

Gonorrhea- Neisseria gonorrhoeae- easy treated.
Males-dysuria, purulent discharge.
Females--discharge, burning urination- find during Pap smear from a squeeze of the Bartholomew gland.
Untreated can lead to sterility-ascending scar tissue make narrow urethra.

HIV-Western Blot
Mild viral illness initial infection- like flu symptoms.
Reverse Transcriptase RNA and Protease Inhibitors stops move from RNA to DNA.
Take combination medications as scheduled.
Terminal Illness.
If caught early take drugs better chance to live longer if missed dose take as soon as you can.

Syphilis
Primary-3-8 weeks-very contagious small sore.
Chancre-HA, lymph enlargement
Secondary-contagious- systematic changes easy treated with penicillin G in primary and secondary stages.
Headache, sore throat, hair loss, arthritis
Tertiary-1-20 years after infection- incurable, will get arthritis, neuropathy and will die.
Systemic, no cure, not contagious

Menstrual Disorders:

Dysmenorrhea–painful menstruation.
Amenorrhea–absence of menstruation. Not uncommon for athletes or under 16.
Polymenorrhea-menstrual cycles of less than 21 days.
 First will try birth control to correct.
Oligomenorrhea–diminished menstrual flow that is not amenorrhea.
Interventions based on cause of disorder.

Contraception "The Pill"

Prevent ovulation
Increased Thickness of cervical mucous makes resistant to sperm penetration.
Endometrium less hospitable if fertilized ovum arrives.
Caution-consult doctor if bleeding, CVA, history of breast cancer, smoker over 35, anticonvulsants and birth control are questionable.

Oral Contraceptives

Regular & extended cycle
Side Effects - nausea, headache, breast tenderness, weight gain, spotting, amenorrhea.
Nurse care Education – how to take the drug, when, pull out insert and go over side effects.

Hormone Implants & Injections

Norplant's - 6 match like capsules of progesterone placed in upper arm.
Big complaint periods not regular. Surgical implant and removed.
Great for latex allergy patients.
Problems- head aches and still have periods and mood swings.
100% effectiveness approximately Last 5 years. Can be removed at anytime.

Depo-Provera-slow release progesterone last 3 months.
Give 5 days after menstruation or 6 weeks after breast feeding well established.
Intrauterine Devices (IUD)

ParaGard-T shaped
Plastic contains copper effective approximately 10 years always check the cord. Causes irritation to uterine wall.

Progestasert-T shape
Contains progesterone in stem: replace yearly 98% effective
Difference -Diaphragm must re measure after each child or 10 lb of weight gain or loss.

Barrier Methods
Blocks entrance of the cervix
Spermicidal foam or suppository. Male/Female condoms available.

Natural Family Planning
Abstinence-100% effective.
Rarely an option -sexuality adds to the quality of life.
Support among religious groups for unmarried couples and adolescents.
Requires extensive assessment and attention to details.
High failure rate - >20%

Types of Natural Family Planning:
Basal Body Temperature
Basal temp rise (0.4) at ovulation
Rise in temp last 14 days indicate pregnancy.
Better at predicting when pregnancy has occurred.

Rhythm Method
Keep track of cycles 14 days on 28 day cycle-16 days on a 30 day cycle. Cervical mucus changes are monitored for determining when ovulation_occurs through the cervical mucus monitoring test. As your cycle progresses, your cervical mucus increases in volume and changes texture. The changes in the mucus that is secreted from the cervix reflect where you are in your cycle. The consistency of your cervical mucus changes during the cycle due to hormonal fluctuations. You are considered most fertile when the mucus becomes clear, slippery, and stretchy. Test with litmus paper to test for PH.

Sterilization
Male vasectomy can be reversed
Female -tubal ligation
Almost 100% effective
Permanent - in some cases can be reversed.

Chapter 9

Complications of Pregnancy Review

Effects and Complications of Pregnancy
External Factors that Affect the Fetus.
Maternal Disease- preexisting conditions, rubella, hypertension.
Use of Drugs, Alcohol, Caffeine, Cigarettes.
Exposure to pollutants
Exposure to radiation
Folic acid for /neurotubule.
Maternal Nutrition –increase calorie 300 day, 500 if lactation, calcium 1200mg day, protein 10mg day.

Factors Affecting Psychological Response:
Body image- take care of them self.
Financial situation- WIC
Cultural expectations
Emotional security- knowing your family supports you.
Support from significant others.

Common Terms
Parity-number of births, not the number of fetuses past 20 weeks, dead or alive.
Hegar's Sign- 6 wks softening of uterus.
Goodell's Sign- 2 month-softening of cervix.
Chadwick's Sign-blue coloration of mucous membranes, vulva, vagina, cervix.
Linea nigra-abdomen
Striae gravidarum-stretch marks.
Prenatal- before birth
Ante partum-before
Postpartum- after
Pseudocyesis- false pregnancy.
Primigravida-pregnant for the first time.
Multigravida-2+ pregnancy.
Gravida-a pregnant woman- Gravidity-number of pregnancies.

Nulligravida- never been pregnant.
Chloasma-pigmentation, face, breast, abdomen.
Colostrum-pre milk
Trimester- 3 months
Quickening-as early as 14-16 wks- fetal movement.
Ballottement-rebounding of the fetus against the examiners finger on palpitation.
Braxton Hicks contractions- irregular, painless.

Reproduction System Changes
Uterus
Cervix
Ovaries
Vagina
Breasts

Cardiovascular Changes
Blood flow increases.
Heart rate increases.
Blood pressure decreases.
Supine hypotensive syndrome may occur.
Physiologic anemia of pregnancy may occur.

Respiratory Changes
Progesterone decreases airway resistance.
The enlarging uterus presses upward on the diaphragm.
Estrogen causes edema and vascular congestion in the nasal mucosa.

Muscular skeletal Changes
Relaxin relaxes the pelvic joints.
Mother's center of gravity changes.
May cause the woman to have a waddling gait.

Gastrointestinal Changes
Nausea and/or vomiting common before 12 weeks.
Delayed gastric emptying and decreased peristalsis.
Stomach and intestines are displaced.
Constipation and heartburn also common.

Urinary Changes
Enlarging uterus presses on bladder in first and third trimester.
Ureters relax and dilate.
Glomerular filtration rate rises.
Glycosuria may develop if kidneys are unable to reabsorb glucose.

Integumentary Changes
Several skin pigment changes occur.
Linea nigra–pigmented line on the abdomen from umbilicus to pubis.
Chloasma–the "mask of pregnancy"
Striae gravidarum– "stretch marks."

Endocrine Changes
Prolactin is responsible for initial milk production.
Oxytocin causes uterine contractions and ejection of milk from the breasts. Also in nasal spray.
Greater insulin production is required.
Thyroid often increases in size.

Metabolism Changes
The metabolic rate of the mother increases during pregnancy as demands of the growing fetus increase.
Mother must meet her own and the fetus' nutritional needs.

Possible Signs of Pregnancy
Amenorrhea
Nausea and vomiting
Breast changes
Urinary frequency
Excessive fatigue
Abdominal enlargement
Quickening

Probable Signs of Pregnancy
Goodell's sign
Hegar's sign
Chadwick's sign
Uterine enlargement

Braxton-Hicks contractions
Increased pigmentation
Ballottement

Pregnancy Test
Measures hCG in either urine or blood.
Blood is positive 8 days after conception.
Urine is positive 10–14 days after conception.
A pregnancy test is a probable sign of pregnancy.

Positive Signs of Pregnancy
Hearing the fetal heartbeat.
Visualization of the fetus through ultrasound.
Examiner feeling fetal movement.

Calculating Estimate Date of Confinement
Nägele's Rule
1st day of last menstrual period (LMP)+7 days minus 3 mos.+1 year.
Sonogram method: Measurement of gestational sac, crown to rump
or crown to heel length.

Prenatal Care
Healthy, prepared mother, minimal discomforts.
Potential problems or complications Identified as early as possible.
Safe delivery of a healthy infant
Prepared father, partner
Prepared siblings and grandparents

Nursing Diagnoses
Activity intolerance
Anxiety
Breathing pattern, ineffective
Body image disturbance
Constipation
Fatigue, or Disturbed sleep pattern
Family coping
Fear

Fetal Well Being Assessment
Ultrasound
Non-stress test
Fetal acoustic stimulation test and vibroacoustic stimulation test.
Fetal biophysical profile, Fetal movements
Biochemical assessments
Amniocentesis
Chorionic villi sampling
Contraction stress test
External fetal monitoring
Internal fetal monitoring

Frequently Occurring Complications during Pregnancy
Hyperemesis Gravidarum-excessive vomiting.
Hydatidiform mole- vaginal bleed like prune juice and have all signs of pregnancy. High risk for cancer.
Placenta Previa- upper 3rd posterior is normal area for placenta.
Abruptio placenta- extreme pain
Polyhydramnios
Oligohydramnios
Ectopic Pregnancy outside of uterus.

Hyperemesis Gravidarum
Excessive vomiting during pregnancy.
Treatment: control vomiting, correct dehydration, restore electrolyte balance, and maintain adequate nutrition.

Hydatidiform Mole
Abnormality of placenta—chorionic villi become fluid-filled, grapelike clusters.
Classic signs are bleeding, uterine enlargement, no fetal heart tones, and hyperemesis,
Gravidarum or symptoms of pregnancy-induced hypertension appear before 24 weeks.
The primary diagnostic tool is ultrasound.
The mole is removed surgically. The client must be followed for 1 to 2 years to monitor for metastasis.

Bleeding Disorders of Late Pregnancy
Placenta Previa
Characterized by painless vaginal bleeding, usually bright red.
No vaginal examination.
Increased risk of infection or hemorrhage after birth.
Cesarean delivery done for partial or total placenta previa.

Abruptio Placenta
Premature separation from wall of uterus of a normally implanted placenta. Symptoms include a rigid, painful abdomen.
Irreversible brain damage or fetal death may occur if hypoxia is not reversed quickly.

Ectopic Pregnancy
Occurs when a fertilized ovum implants outside the uterine cavity.
The most common site is fallopian tube.
Pain is noted as the tube stretches with the growing embryo, eventually rupturing.
Rapid surgical treatment is generally necessary to control bleeding.

Disseminated Intravascular Coagulation (DIC)
Overstimulation of normal clotting process occurs as complication of a primary problem.
It can cause fetal death.
Symptom onset sudden: dyspnea, chest pain, restlessness, cyanosis, and spitting frothy, blood-tinged mucous.
Underlying cause must be identified and corrected.
The fetus must be delivered.
Pregnancy Induced Hypertension PIC = HELP/Hemolysis/elevated liver enzymes/low platelets.
Most common hypertensive disorder in pregnancy, after 20 weeks' gestation.
Only cure is delivery of the baby.
Mild preeclampsia—blood pressure increases 30 mm Hg systolic or 15 mm Hg diastolic over.
baseline on two occasions at least 6 hours apart.

Edema noted in face and hands.
Objectively defined as weight gain of more than 1 pound a week.
Urine may show 1+ or 2+ albumin.
Proteinuria usually the last of the three classic symptoms to appear.
Severe preeclampsia–blood pressure increases to 160/110 or higher.
Generalized edema in face, hands, sacral area, lower extremities, and abdomen.
Weight gain may be 2 pounds a week.
Urinary albumin may be 3+ or 4+.

Other symptoms: continuous headache, blurred vision, scotomata, nausea, vomiting, irritability, hyperreflexia, and epigastric pain.
Epigastric pain often last symptom identified before client moves into eclampsia.
Eclampsia–grand mal seizures.
Without treatment, the client may die.
Treat to lower blood pressure, prevent convulsions, and deliver a healthy baby.
Magnesium sulfate given to prevent convulsions.

Magnesium Sulfate- to prevent convulsions.
Respirations must be at least 14/minute.
Deep tendon reflexes must be kept at normal response.
Urine output must be at least 30 cc/hour.
Monitor serum magnesium level.
Calcium gluconate is antidote for magnesium sulfate–keep at bedside.

Diabetes Mellitus
Diabetic clients: disease under control.
Gestational diabetes mellitus appears only during pregnancy.
Pregnancy in a diabetic client has a higher risk of complications.
Macrosomia, excessive fetal growth, results from maternal hyperglycemia.

Chronic Hypertension
BP 140/90 or higher before pregnancy or before the 20th week of gestation that lasts longer than 6 weeks after delivery.

Clients with moderate to severe chronic hypertension are most at risk to develop PIH.

Heart Disease

Normal physiological changes of pregnancy may cause problems in client with heart disease.

Many clients are cared for by both their cardiologist and obstetrician.

Antibiotics often used as a prophylaxis for all pregnant women with heart disease.

Maternal Phenylketonuria-law to test baby for PKU at birth.

When woman with PKU keeps her phenylalanine level less than 2.0 mg/dl while pregnant,

Outcome of pregnancy better.

The mother's blood phenylalanine level should be checked throughout pregnancy.

Client to maintain phenylalanine-free diet.

Torch Group of Infections.

Toxoplasmosis (TO)-bacteria kitty litter, eats baby brain.

Rubella (R) - while pregnant, baby can or will be blind, deaf.

Cytomegalovirus (C) - kidneys of fetus.

Herpes genitalis (H) - ascending bacteria- attacks spinal fluid.

If untreated: abortion, congenital anomalies, fetal infections, IUGR, preterm labor, mental Retardation, death.

HIV/AIDS- no breastfeeding. Weight gain is a challenge for pregnant HIV-infected client.

HIV may be transmitted to fetus through placenta, during birth, or during breast feeding.

Nutritional counseling and support may be necessary.

Hemolytic Diseases Rh incompatibility–can only happen when mother is Rh negative and fetus is Rh positive.

ABO incompatibility–problem occurs when maternal blood enters fetal circulation.

RhoGAM is a byproduct of blood and will get the antibodies. Rh.

Multiple Pregnancies
First trimester precedes much the same as with a single fetus.
As uterus grows greater pressure on and displacement of the internal organs.
Greater risk of fetal anomalies, abnormal presentations, and preterm birth.

Substance Abuse
Substance abusers may not seek prenatal care until late in pregnancy.
Most do not voluntarily admit addiction.
These mothers have an increased rate of complications.
They often use available money for drugs instead of food.

Preterm Labor
Labor that begins after viability but before 38 weeks' gestation.
Causes maternal, fetal, or placental.
Preterm labor may produce a neonate not able to cope well with extrauterine life.
The process of stopping labor with medications is called tocolysis.
Shirodkar Procedure - Incompetent Cervix.

Cues for Post-partum Assessment-BUBBLE-HE
B-Breast
U-Uterus
B-Bladder
B-Bowel
L-Lochia
E-Episiotomy
H-Homan's Sign
E-Emotional State

Cues for Assessing Incision Sites-REEDA
R-Redness
E-Edema
E-Ecchymosis
D-Drainage
A-Accomodation

Lochia rubra – bright red, blood till 3-4 days PP-Post Partum.
Lochia serosa - brown, old blood tissue debris can last up to 22-27 days PP
Lochia Alba – yellow white, leukocytes, mucus lasts up to 6 weeks PP, starts about 10 days PP in most women.
Pitocin – contractions of uterus, decreases bleeding, monitor vaginal bleeding and uterine tone.

Chapter 10

Newborns and Congenital Malformations

The Newborn at Risk & Appearances.
Preterm less than 37 weeks-Term 38 – 40 weeks-Post Term, more than 40 weeks.
SGA-below 10% regardless of gestation.
LGA-weight above 90 %
IUGR-Growth retarded
AGA-Appropriate for gestational age.

Perinatal Factors that place infant at risk
Maternal health history-mom who has heath problems.
Complications of Pregnancy or Labor-PIH, gestational diabetes.
Size & Gestation Age
Difficulty of Birth- dystocia or prolapse cord or O2.
Narcotic administration within 1 – 1½ hour of birth.
Precipitous-fast delivery

Thermoregulation
Evaporation – parents bathing infant slowly.
Conduction – infant placed on cool padded surface for assessment.
Convection – Air-conditioning vent blowing air on infant.
Radiation – Infant's crib located near window on a cold day.
Brown Fat Location-at term- kidneys, on back of neck and scapula-lose 10 % of this fat right away.

Methods to Reduce Hypothermia
Drying – reduces evaporation heat lost.
Hat – reduces heat loss through the head-Head is 25% percent of skin surface-Apply to dry head do not use under warmer.
Radiant Warmer – adds supplemental heat.
Parent contact – Skin to skin warming- Kangaroo care, body to body to keep warm.

Umbilical Cord

Umbilical cord-finger breath above umbilicus.

Three vessels- 2 Arteries – carries blood away from baby- 1Large Vein – carries blood and nutrients to baby.

Vessels supported by Wharton's Jelly- keeps from kinks.

Normal length-12 to 36 inches or (30 to 90 cm)

Vitamin K- Aqua- Mephyton

Newborns have temp. Deficiency in Vitamin. K

For formation of clotting factors manufactured by bacteria in the intestines. Needs to eat to form bacteria.

Intestinal tract is temporary. Sterile at birth until normal flora is established, must have food to produce bacteria.

Always given intramuscular in the anterior thigh 0.5 to 1 mg 5lb or less 0.5mg.

Ophthalmia Neonatorum-purulent conjunctivitis & keratitis of newborn eyes from exposure to gonorrhea and chlamydia. Public health department requires all infants be treated with erythromycin ophthalmic ointment following birth- leave in 1 minute, signs of infection must be cultured. Parents can sign a waiver.

Fontanelle- allows brain to grow

Anterior-Diamond Shape 2 parietal bones & 2 frontal bones Closes at 12 to 18 months.

Posterior-Triangular in Shape 2 parietal bones & one occipital bone closes by end of 2nd month.

Function: allow head to adapt to diameter of the birth canal & allow for future growth.

Craniostenosis- fontanel's closed- surgery to open to allow brain to grow.

Vital Signs

Apnea: more than 15 seconds: not uncommon: count for one full minute.

Heart Rate – 2 types of murmurs frequently heard.

Functional: is normal and due to blood passing through the nl heart valves.

Organic: due to abnormal openings or nl openings that have not closed yet.

Temperature: Initial is usually rectal then axillary-Lubricate – insert 0.5 inches.

Musculoskeletal Assessment

Movements are random and uncoordinated.

Eyes often appear cross-eyed –nystagmus normal.

Tremors during crying are normal. Constant tremors during sleep may not be normal.

Muscle tone – should not be limp- would be signs of cardiac or hyperglycemia.

Newborn's Kidney Function

Blood flow - ⅓ of adult renal blood flow-1cc per kg per hour.

Reabsorption functions:

Short renal tubules limit capacity to reabsorb substances.

Glucose, amino acids, phosphates, bicarbonate- insufficient surfactant.

Limited ability to concentrate urine.

Limited ability to cope with fluid imbalances.

Fontanel's sink in if dehydrated- should be flat also mucus membranes will be dry and skin turgor.

Circumcision

Yellen or Gomco – Plastibell- never use Vaseline on this one, bell is put on and tied skin necrosis and falls off.

Pros-Prevention of premature CA, Fewer UTI's-Decrease in transmission of STD's.

Cons-Hemorrhage & infection.

AAP- (American academy of pediatrics) do not support circumcision-Cosmetic and Strictly parental choice.

Newborn Stools

Meconium: green/ black, thick and sticky passed 8 – 24° after birth.

Transitional: loose and green/yellow, contain mucus usually gone 1st week.

Breastfed infants stool: yellow soft and pasty may have 3 to 6 per day or every time they feed.
Bottle fed: yellow/brown, more solid and fewer in numbers.
Abnormal stools:
Small putty-like-liver problems.
Diarrhea
Bloody stool- possible fissure if bright red is on outside of stool, do cultures to be sure for fetal or maternal blood.

Feeding Infants- 120 cal per kg per day.
Forms of Formula: ready to feed single use, ready to feed cans, concentrated liquid, and powder.
Never prop a bottle
Do not heat in microwave
Discard leftover formula- most 4 hours.
Position on back or side

Newborn Screening
PKU – mandatory in every state- build up of PKU- control by diet, causes retardation- most blonde blue eyed.
Hypothyroidism-cause growth failure- can take Synthroid rest of life.
Galactosemia-intolerance of lactose (milk sugar) - special diet.
Sickle cell disease- transfusion- interferes with carry of O2.
Thalassemia-polypeptide chain deficiency of alpha and beta production.
Maple Syrup Urine Disease- metabolism- amino acids-urine smells sweet..plus 32 other test.

Jaundice
Normal occurrence. Excess RBCs are destroyed after birth because baby breaths air and get oxygen directly.
The high Hct (large number of erythrocytes) is unnecessary after birth. Appears 2 to 3 days after birth last about 7 days- direct sun works great if in range.
Treatment: Based on levels bilirubin less than 25, phototherapy, mask only, blanket therapy don't need goggle's.

Discharge Instructions
Rest
Hygiene
Sexual intercourse
Exercise
Diet
Nine danger signals that the PP mom needs to report immediately.

Assessing Gestational Age and The Premature Infant
Respiratory (RDS) - fast breathing- tachypnea.
Decreased Surfactant-produce their own 28 wks.
Circulation-ductus arteriosus reopens, get anemia- will have wide blood pressure.
GI-NPO-TPN for 21 days.
Metabolic- cannot produce glucose- hypoglycemic.
IVH- interventricular hemorrhage- ventricles bleed in brain.
Renal- not developed, no gravity, common to see protein in urine.
Immune System-no IgG, cough into shoulder to prevent spread of germs.
Nutrition-TPN, can't handle high proteins.
Appearance- transparent skin looks old.
Parents unable to care for infant- involve mom /dad.
Loss of perfect child- want Gerber baby.
Emotional needs back n forth to hospital.
Common reactions- what they did wrong.

Post Term infant
Long and thin as if weight loss has occurred.
Loss skin especially around thighs and buttocks.
Skin dry & cracks easily, parchment like skin- like peel it off.
Long dagger like nails- never cut nail without permission of doctor, maybe culture issue.

Environmental Needs
Isolette
Radiant Warmers
Temperature & Humidity

Oxygen- not how much O2 are getting -how muchO2 is on blood can cause blindness, laser surgery for this.
Observation- skin, noise, color, sleepy (ABC) don't do blood pressure unless suspect cardio problem (systolic 60)
Nursing Care- VS per protocol.

SGA-Can be Preterm, term, post term.
Decreased amount of adipose tissue.
Symmetrical – smaller in all three parameters- head, chest, length.
Asymmetrical – average head circumference 13-14mm – large head 15 ok within limits.

LGA-May be Preterm, term, post term.
Birth weight 4000 g (8 lbs 14½ oz.)
Large parents have large babies.
Native Americans are more likely to have LGA infants- genetics.
Shoulder dystocia.
Fracture of the clavicle.
Brachial plexus palsies.
Depressed skull fractures.
Cephalohematoma- does not cross suture line. Capitus S (fluid) does cross suture line.
Passage of meconium in utero.

Diseases of the Infant at Risk
Retinopathy of Prematurity- scar tissue in retina.
Respiratory Distress Syndrome- if mom is diabetic.
Hemolytic Diseases- ABO do Coombs test to test for incompatible.
Hyperbilirubinemia
Hypo & Hyperglycemia
Neonatal Sepsis

Hypo & Hyperglycemia-Insufficient store of glycogen & fat.
Any condition increases use of these stores.
Plasma glucose levels <40 mg/dl
120 – 150 kcal/Kg/day to grow 100 just to maintain.
S&S:-Tremors, Weak cry, Lethargy, convulsion.

Congenital Malformation

Hydrocephalus

Noncommunicating-Obstructive-Prevents flow from ventricles of the brain to the subarachnoid space- surgery.

Communicating-CSF inadequately reabsorbed in the subarachnoid space- shunt behind ear goes to peritoneal cavity.

Nursing Care

Pre-op-Frequent repositioning to prevent pressure ulcers.

Nutritional support.

Post-op

Observe for ICP

High pitch cry, unequal pupil size, irritability.

Lethargy, poor feeding.

Care of the Shunt- position on opposite side, balloon must be soft.

Encephalocele

Herniation of part of the brain from the cranial cavity – may contain CSF as well as brain tissue.

Spina Bifida_-Imperfect closure of the spinal vertebrae-1st 6 wks of conception.

Elevated AFP levels- alpha fetoprotein.

Occulta- Small opening no protrusion of structures- hair patch.

Cystic mass in the midline of the spine.

Two Types:

Meningocele – contains a portion of membranes and CSF.

Meningomyelocele – contains membranes, spinal cord.

Cleft Lip & Cleft Palate

Pre-op care-Nutrition- breast feed or special bottles.

Post-op care-Preventing dislodging sutures- restrain hands-Care of appliances – wash between feedings.

Cleft lip- complete/ incomplete (doesn't go up to nares.

Cleft palate-soft palate only- unilateral/bilateral complete- surgery at 6 months.

Dislocation of the Hip and Talipes Equinovarus (Club Foot)
Assessment done visually by nurse.
Slings and diapers.
Occasionally require surgery.
Ortolani's – relocates- pop in.
Barlow's – dislocates- pop out.
Cast care – Shoes.
Parental support.

Down Syndrome-Most common Genetic Disorder.
Nondisjunction – failure to follow nl separation process- lots of problems mental retardation.
Mosaicism – nondisjunction occurs late in development.
Translocation – a piece of 21 breaks away & attaches on another chromosome.
Trisomy 21-Close set upward slanting eyes- most common 21st chromosome has 3.
Small head - round face.
Protruding tongue.
Mental retardation.
Limp flaccid posture.

Metabolic Disorders -Autosomal recessive trait= among sexes.

PKU – phenylketonuria-Deficiency of the enzyme phenylalanine hydroxylase found in the liver.
Test ideally done at 3 – 4 days of age.
Phenylalanine > 25 mg/dl (normal <2mg/dl) only 5% of positive test have PKU.
Treatment: low-phenylalanine diet. ** avoid NutraSweet as it converts to PKU usually uses Lofenalac for formula.

Maple Syrup Urine Disease (MSUD) Disorder of the metabolism of leucine, Isoleucine and valine.
Occurs in the liver.
Treatment- started in first 10 days.
Diet low in branch chain amino-acids.

Galactosemia-Autosomal recessive disorder of galactose metabolism.
Galactose is disaccharide lactose synthesized from glucose.
Deficiency in galactokinase.
Untreated develop cataracts.
Galactose - glucose is present in milk, body cannot use carbohydrates = galactose glucose.

Chapter 11

Endocrine System Review

Where do hormones come from? Hypothalamus, pituitary, thyroid, parathyroid.
Pituitary, thyroid, parathyroid, adrenal, teste, ovary, pancreas (isle of Langerhans)
Pancreas- produces insulin. Insulin is needed for transport of glucose into the cell.
Normal glucose level 70-115. Insulin pump patient doesn't change the lifestyle, as pump is set for their daily activities.

Causes and Prevention
Imbalance of hormones-over or under secretions.

Diagnostic Tests
Lab Tests-levels of hormones for each organ- Calcium (parathyroid) major role.
MRI
CAT Scans
Scans-Iodine uptake (thyroid) radioactive isotope.

Nursing Process
Assessment weight gain, or loss, tired, nausea, constipation, voice change.
-history insomnia, heart palpitations, temp change, hair change, dry scale skin.
-physical vital signs, hair, nails, do they look tired.

Nursing Diagnoses
Body Image Disturbance
Fatigue
Sleep pattern disturbance
Risk for infection
Risk for injury

Pituitary Gland

Normal Function-it is the master gland.
Hormones-LH, FSH, GH, ACTH, TSH
Diagnostic Tests -hormone levels.
LH Luteinizing hormone.
FSH follicular stimulant hormone.
GH growth hormone
ACTH adrenocorticotropic hormone.
TSH Thyroid stimulant hormone. Pituitary to thyroid T3-T4.

Tumors

-depends upon size.
-Small--vague and generalized.
-Large-head ache and visual disturbance.
-Location of tumor- Acromegaly-excessive GH
Treatment-replace hormones- Surgery-removal of tumor and/or radiation.

Diabetes Insipidus

ADH
Copious amounts of urine.

Syndrome of Inappropriate Antidiuretic Hormone (SIADH)-

Excessive production ADH.
S & S-confusion, seizures, weight gain and edema.
Treatment- treat underlying cause; fluid restriction, Diuretics.
Thyroid-Normal Function-metabolism- protein and lipid synthesis.
Diagnostic Tests and Procedures-T3, T4.
-Iodine Uptake
-Scan

Goiter-Enlargement of Thyroid.
S & S-early-enlargement in front of neck.
Later-difficulty swallowing/breathing.
Treatment- iodine or iodized salt.-will not cure the problem.-surgical removal.

Hyperthyroidism-Primary-thyroid (Grave's Disease) Bug Eyes.
-elevated T3 triiodothyronine and T4 thyroxin.
Secondary-pituitary
-elevated TSH
-accelerated metabolic rate.
-weight loss, insomnia, tachycardia, difficulty concentration, scant menstruation, decreased libido.
Treatment-Radioactive iodine (131 I)-SSKI
Nursing Interventions-high caloric intake, adequate rest.

Hypothyroidism- Lack of thyroid hormone, Inflammation.
Hyperthyroidism, genetic; myxedema (low production)
-reduced metabolism
-lethargic, excessive sleeping, weight gain, inability to concentrate, sluggish mentally and physically.
-increased sensitivity to cold, rough dry skin, non pitting edema.
Treatment-Replacement of hormones.
Nursing Interventions
-do not rush, lotion for skin, extra warmth, psychosocial aspects.
-do not stop meds.
-monitor for Myxedema Coma.
-loss of consciousness, B/P, RR, T, hypoglycemia.
-airway management, glucose, corticosteroids, fluids.

Thyroidectomy-removal of 2/3
-Tracheostomy set at bedside a must.
-Fowler's Semi
Vital signs and observe for an increase in temperature, pulse, respiration rate and, hoarseness.

Thyroid crisis (storm) from removal of thyroid.
Excess thyroxine R/T related to; manipulation.
Extreme elevation of all body process
Tempurature-106; Paulse-200 bpm; Respiration Rate.-30-40.
-extreme restlessness/apprehension.

Tetany- Usually manipulation or accidental removal of parathyroid responsible for Ca in muscles.
Medical Emergency.
Muscle cramping, twitching, convulsions.
IV Calcium Gluconate in crisis.
Parathyroid hormone for maintenance.

Parathyroid-Normal Function-regulates calcium levels.
Diagnostic Tests
-parathormone levels
-Calcium levels

Hypoparathyroid (Von Recklinghausen's Disease)
-Hypercalcemia
S & S-dehydration, confusion, lethargy, anorexia, nausea, vomiting, weight loss,
constipation, thirst, polyuria, hypertension, Osteoporosis.
Treatment-NaCl, Diuretics, Phosphate, Mithramycin (inhibit skeletal release of calcium)

Adrenal Glands
Normal Function
-medulla
-epinephrine and norepinephrine
-cortex
Mineralocorticoid (Aldosterone)
Glucocorticoids (Hydrocortisone)
Androgenic hormones

Addison's disease
Decrease of adrenal cortex-vital signs everything goes down.
Involves hormones (androgenic compensation in ovaries and testes)
S & S-imbalances (hyponatremia and hyperkalemia); muscle weakness and pain; hypotension. Anorexia, nausea, vomiting, diarrhea, loss of mental acuity; hypoglycemia.
Treatment-Hormone replacement
Inborn Errors of Metabolism-Hundreds of hereditary biochemical disorders that affect metabolism-Generally autosomal recessive.

Tay - Sachs disease -autosomal recessive-Missing enzyme necessary for fat metabolism- Lipid deposits accumulate on nerve cells. Children- normal until 5-6 mos.-Physical development slows, large head/Inability to sit- Mental retardation - Blindness may occur. - Death occurs usually by age 5.

Endocrine Disorders large heads tongue stuck out, large umbilical hernia.*can live normal life if meds are given.
Hypothyroidism-Deficiency in secretions of thyroid gland-Congenital or Juvenile acquired.
-One of the more common endocrine problems in children.
Treatment-Medication, Regular evaluation of T4 TSH for dosing adjustments.
If untreated severe irreversible, mental retardation & physical difficulties continue.

Diabetes Insipidus-Hereditary (autosomal dominant) or Acquired (head injury or tumor)-kidney does not concentrate urine. Decreased Secretion of vasopressin (antidiuretic hormone)
Initial **S/S** polyuria, polydipsia.
-Monitor for signs of over-dosage-Edema, lethargy, nausea CNS signs.
Need medical ID band/ inform schools of your child's condition.

Type I, Insulin Dependent Diabetes Mellitus (IDDM) -Chronic metabolic condition.
Unable to use CHO properly. **Type I**-juvenile-IDDM-insulin dependent Lack of insulin all the way.
Glucose floats around but cells cannot absorb into cell. Loose muscle mass.
Need insulin in order for the cell to absorb glucose. Starts in young people.
Show more symptoms and also can have increased sugar. Can die of Ketoacidosis.

Type II

adult onset-NIDDM-non insulin dependent. Does not get Ketoacidosis. The problem is long term effect. Will not die because of increased sugar. Usually found in routine checkups. 50 years of age, lifestyles, obesity are factors.

Pancreas does not produce enough insulin so insulin by mouth is administered and will eventually progress to injections.

Deficiency of insulin * make sure kids know the life long illness is all about.

-Impairment of glucose transport

-Body cannot store or use fats properly.

-Decrease in protein synthesis

Autoimmune disease-Chromosome number 6- Most common endocrine disorder in children.

Differences between Adult Onset & Juvenile Diabetes

Juvenile- Primarily in childhood- Insulin dependent- Usually weight loss *7 year old can do own insulin.

Adult-Usually after 40 yrs-Non-insulin dependent- Usually obese.

DM more severe in Children

Growing- Expanded energy needs, Nutritional needs vary.

Must face a lifetime of diabetic management.

Symptoms in Children-3 P's:

Polyuria-excretions of large amounts of urine.

Polydipsia-Excessive thirst.

Polyphagia-Excessive hunger *know these signs.

Fatigue, Anorexia, Nausea, Lethargy & weakness.

Dry skin. Vaginal yeast infection. Bedwetting in trained child.

Medical Management

Blood/Urine Values

FBS (> 180mg/dL)

Insulin levels

Urine glucose levels

Glycosylated hemoglobin test.

Nursing interventions

Educational Needs: Injection site rotation-Self administration around 7 years of age.

Nutritional-Distribute food intake so that it aids metabolic control-Individualize diet to:

Age, sex, weight, activity, ethnic background, economics and food preferences.

Regular meals & snacks.

Sports Activity-Check blood sugars hourly

Watch for dry mouth and eyes.

Drop in blood sugar need a source of sugar, protein and starch with them.

Foot Care- change socks and shoes.

Traveling need to have-Orange juice, regular soda + protein & starch.

Hypoglycemia

Caused by insulin excess-Sudden onset in healthy child.

Blood sugar < 55mg/dL, intestinal surgery, pancreas stressors, liver, and endocrine.

Initial symptoms-Sweating, tremor, feeling cold, anxiety, hunger.

Late symptoms-Confusion, weakness, dizziness, nausea, vomiting headache, stupor, convulsions.

At Risk-Alcoholics and Drug Addicts.

Diagnosis-GTT (glucose tolerance test)

Treatment diet-complex sugars, high protein, frequent meals, medication.

Hypoglycemia in Newborn-Low blood sugar.

Abrupt decrease in maternal glucose.

Hypertrophy of pancreatic islet cells.

FBS < 40 mg/dL

Cushingoid appearance increased subcutaneous fat.

Immature, RDS, congenital anomalies-Severe SGA or poor placental perfusion-Hypoglycemic, hypocalcemic, hyperbilirubinemia.

Nursing Care
Close monitoring of Vital signs.
Blood sugars on infants weighing over 9 lbs or fewer than 6 pounds
(Check with facility)
Early feedings (some issue with breast feedings)
Observe for signs of irritability, tremors.
If untreated may result in permanent brain damage.

Ketoacidosis-Caused by insulin deficiency-(severe hyperglycemia)
Appears over hours or days
Blood sugar more than 200 mg/dL
Ketonuria
Initial symptoms-Thirst, dry skin, abdominal pain, flushed-Restless,
fruity odor to breath.
Late symptoms-Acidosis, dehydration, Kussmaul breathing, coma.

Infants of Diabetic Mother
Degree depends on severity & duration of mother's condition.
Degree of control & gestational age-When control- minimal affects
on infant.
Hyperglycemic moms transfer large amounts of glucose to fetus.
Fetal pancreas produce large amounts of insulin (Hyperinsulinism)
As well as excess production of protein fatty acids- LGA.
Prone to birth trauma - macrosomia.

Somogyi & Dawn Phenomenon-Most common causes of
instability in diabetic children.
Somogyi-Rebound hyperglycemia—blood sugar testing all night long
to determine Somogyi or Dawn.
*need to do a 3am Blood stick.
-Glucose released from muscle and liver cells.
-Results from chronic insulin use esp. large doses.
-Hypoglycemic during night-hyperglycemia in am.
Dawn-early morning elevations of blood glucose occur without
preceding hypoglycemia.
May be response to growth hormone release.
Test at 3 am helps to differentiate the two.

Diabetes Review Contributing Factors
Genetics-(1)
Stress
Emotional
Physical
Obesity- (2) high sugar diet, lifestyle.
Viral- (1) viral infection
Autoimmune-(1)
S &S- tingling and numbness on feet.
3 P's- (1)
Polydipsia-glucose ↑osmotic pressure and drink water, glucose spills
out in urine.
Keystones in urine is byproduct of protein
Polyuria
Polyphagia
Fatigue and weakness- (1) and (2)
Weight-up (2) or down (1)
Slow healing infections

Diagnostic Tests
FBS-NPO at midnight
FSBS-finger stick
Urine-sugar and ketones
GTT-glucose tolerant test- take FBS then drink syrup two hours later
will take another test, blood sugar should be normal.
2 hour postprandial- measure Blood sugar 2 hr after meals and
should be in normal range.
Glycosylated Hemoglobin (A1c)-routine lab, don't have to NPO.
This test tells how they have been behaving for the last 3 months.
4.9-6.7% excellent, 7.6-8.5% good, 9.4-10.0 fair, 12.1-13.0 poor.

Complications
Hyperglycemia- ketoacidosis can die from, look like they are drunk.
Diabetic ketoacidosis. Fruity breath, unsteady gait.
Acetonuria
Somogyi Phenomenon- in night surge of hormones blood sugar
bottoms out they die in their sleep.
Hyperglycemic hyperosmolar nonketotic syndrome (HHNS).

Complications- Short term
Hypoglycemia- from vomiting or overexertion drives blood sugar down.
Hypoglycemic very low is more dangerous than too high.
Tremors-Hunger-Head ache, Diaphoretic, Blurred vision.
Treatment-glucose, Orange juice with sugar in it.
Protein intake-peanut butter on cracker, protein is longer acting in body. Check blood sugar every15 minutes to see the level.

Long Term- keep blood sugar in tact so won't have long term complications.
Cardiovascular Disease- from plaque buildup, sometimes it takes an insult to body before see symptoms of heart disease.
Nephropathy
PVD-peripheral vascular disease.
Neuropathy
Retinopathy

Management
Diet- avoid concentrated sweets and fats- work with patient with counting carbohydrates, try not to deprive within limits.
Exercise- increased glucose uptake & decreased lipids level.
Medication- Close control to decrease long term complications.
Medications- Oral hypoglycemic agents- stimulates pancreas to produce insulin.
Diabinese, Micronase, Glucophage.
Newer hypoglycemics makes cells more sensitive.

Nursing Diagnoses
Altered Nutrition
Knowledge Deficit
Risk for Infection
Risk for Injury
Sexual Dysfunction
Ineffective Individual Coping

Insulin- Types- know the peaks for test
Humalog -brand name
Lispro-rapid/very short acting.
Regular- /rapid short acting.
Lente and NPH-intermediate acting.
Mixed- clear before cloudy
70/30-premixed 70 NPH/ 30 R

Insulin Uses
All Type 1 diabetic
Some Type 2 - if not controlled by diet, exercise, oral anti-diabetic meds, or during times of stress and major illness, kidney or liver failure, pregnancy.
Gestational diabetes.
Ketoacidosis, hyperglycemic hyperosmolar nonketotic syndrome.

Onset, Peak, Duration
Using consistent concentration U-100.
Onset - Time from injection, until it begins to lower blood glucose.
Peak - Time from injection until maximum insulin effect.
Duration - Length of time insulin will continue to lower blood glucose.

Ultrashort/Rapid Acting Insulin
Lispro (Humalog) - rapid acting insulin.
Onset is 5 - 15 min, peak 1 - 1.5 hrs, duration 3 - 4hrs.
Need to give within 15 min of food or hypoglycemia can occur.

Lispro (Humalog) or Aspart (NovoLog)
Advantages - meal time flexibility.
Can "dose and eat "take moments before eating, so there's not a problem if meal schedule is irregular.
Especially helpful with kids. Can base dose on how much food the person just consumed.

Humalog Meal Caution

Should eat rapidly absorbed CHO first - liquids, cooked foods, to get into blood stream quickly.

Fat and fiber can delay absorption and cause hypoglycemia.

Regular - "R", pure, unmodified, clear.

Brands - Humulin R, Novolin R.

Administer SC, IM or IV (only insulin that can be given IVP, in IV solution, or drip)

Use to rapidly decrease BG in emergencies (DKA, HHNKS)

Sliding Scale

Manage acute increases in blood glucose on sliding scale - surgery, infection, stress.

Regular Insulin

Use in combination with others (intermediate or long acting) or as sliding scale.

Mimics rapid

Prandial release.

Onset ½ - 1 hr.

Peak 2 - 3 hrs

Duration 4 - 6 hrs

Intermediate-Acting Insulin Cloudy suspensions, (precipitated with protamine and zinc to lengthen duration) administer SC

NPH - "N" and Lente - "L"

Brands – example: Novolin and Humulin

Onset 1-2 hrs, peak 4 or 6-12 hrs, duration 18 to 24 hrs.

May give as single, daily dose or 2 daily doses alone, or mixed with rapid or short-acting.

Start at 10 – 20u, titrates up 4 – 6 u every few days.

Long-acting Insulin

Ultralente, and Humulin U - have broad, flat peak and long duration.

Mimics basal insulin secretion – onset 2 hrs, peak 16 – 20 hrs, duration 24 hrs. May be given in AM as one dose.

May be divided into 2 doses - pre-breakfast, and pre-evening meal, with regular or Humalog.

Prandial increases
Glargine (Lantus) – another brand.
Onset 2 hrs, no peak, duration 24 hrs.
Clear – Danger. Do not mistake for fast/rapid acting insulins.
Do not mix with any other insulin.
Initial dose is 10 u at bedtime, or AM.
Side effect – pain at injection site.

Premixed Insulins
70% NPH / 30% R
50% NPH / 50% R
75% NPH / 25% Humalog
Mimics normal prandial release of insulin (2/3 of total in AM, 1/3 in PM)
Used to mix, now come premixed, much easier for patients.
Best for Type 2.
Can use in insulin pen.

Insulin Pens
Pre-filled (disposable), or
Re-useable pen with cartridge.
Dial turned to set the dose, numbers magnified through window.
Disposable needles. Don't have to: draw up insulin.
More convenient to carry, easier to read.
Available in NPH, 70/30, 75/25, regular, Humalog, Lantus.
More expensive but more convenient.

Chapter 12

Blood Disorders

Lymphatic -Enlarged tonsils and adenoids are normal in preschool and school-age children – body's defense mechanism.
Thymus is important for development of the immune response in newborns.
Spleen is the largest organ of the lymphatic system-enlarges during:
Infections
Congenital and acquired hemolytic anemia.
Liver malfunction

Anemia-Hemoglobin (Hgb) <8 pallor, tachypneic-Results is a decrease in the oxygen carrying capacity of the RBCs. Leads to increased cardiac output and shunting of the blood away from the periphery to the vital organs.
Two common tests performed for blood disorders:
Bone Marrow Aspiration
Blood Counts (CBC with Diff)

Iron Deficiency Anemia-Most common nutritional deficiency of children in the United States.
Incidence highest during infancy (9 to24 months) and adolescence.
Insufficient amounts of iron in blood leads to decrease in size and number of circulating RBCs.
*before 6 months whole milk leads to anemia as body cannot absorb it.
1. Inadequate supply of dietary iron can't form hemoglobin.
2. Impaired absorption of iron received.
3. Blood loss.
4. Excessive demands for iron-growth requirements.
Inability to form hemoglobin.
S&S-Most often not obvious-Common Signs
Over weight/low weight
Paleness
Tachycardia
Positive guaiac test

Poor muscle development
Excessive consumption of milk
Frequently seen
Irritability
Anorexia
Decreased Activity
Murmur
Enlarged spleen
Heart failure can occur from weakened muscle.

Iron Deficiency Anemia
Hgb less than 10, low mean corpuscular volume (MCV) and low mean corpuscular hemoglobin concentration (MCHC), low reticulocyte count.
Fe levels (low serum ferritin)
Fe SO_4 2-3 x/day
Some preparations can discolor teeth.
Vitamin C to aid in absorption."Spooned" nails-sunk in middle high on sides.

Nursing Care -Aim of treatment is to correct cause of anemia.
Dietary counseling
Assess compliance of parent.
Patient/Parent Education-Milk is not the perfect food.
Stools tarry green.
Avoid taking Fe supple with milk or foods high in phosphorus; do not give with Vitamin E supplement.
Avoid Fe poisoning by keeping preparation well out of reach.
*law 'all babies are screened at birth.

Sickle Cell Anemia-Inherited deficiency (autosomal-recessive disorder) in the formation of RBCs. RBCs look like sickle blades (Hgb S)-Have fragile cell membranes-cell life 10-20 days vs. 120 days. Clumping of cells in capillary & small arteries and veins – cells are more rigid and obstruct capillary flow leads to tissue ischemia. Organs become scarred from damaged tissue.
*infections caused by ischemia = leg ulcers less than 6.9 is crisis, swelling of hands and feet.

Sickle Cell Traits-small percentage in African-Americans.
Blood contains a mixture of Hgb A and Hgb S- Hgb S concentration low and is inherited from one parent. Treatment is required but client is a carrier.

Sickle Cell Disease-Severe form of the disease-gene is inherited from both parents.
Symptoms generally do not appear until 4-6 mo of age-Because of the presence of fetal Hgb.

S&S: Ophthalmic-Diminished vision as a result of Vitreous hemorrhage -Retinal Detachment –Blindness.
Brain-headache; convulsion; CVA/by vaso-occlusion of vessels.
Skin- decreased peripheral circulation leading to leg ulcers.
Chest pain, Fever, Cough precipitated by or resulting from pneumonia.
Cardiomegaly-systolic flow murmur.
Abdominal pain
Genitourinary dysfunction (Dilute urine)
Splenic sequestration (pooled blood enlarges spleen)
Bones - painful episodes in joints (arthralgia) & limbs.
Hand & Foot syndrome-symptom of Vaso-occlusion.

Types of Sickle Cell Crisis
Vaso-occlusive: most common typed; painful; -caused by stasis of blood with cell clumping in microcirculation, ischemia, infarction; fever, pain, & tissue engorgement are common signs.
Splenic sequestration: life-threatening crisis; Caused by pooling of blood within spleen.
Anemia, hypovolemia, and shock are common signs.
Aplastic crisis: reduced production & increased destruction of RBCs;- Crisis usually triggered by viral infection.
Anemia & pallor are common signs.

Possible S/S of Crisis-Severe abdominal cramping/pain- Muscle spasms, vomiting, hematuria.
Painful swollen joints, fever, convulsions.

Treatment of Sickle Cell Disease
RBC morphology, Genetic screening
Supportive symptomatic therapy- 1-4 can have it if they carry the gene. Doesn't mean kids will have it.
Blood transfusions
PCN
Pain Meds

Factors That May Trigger Crisis
Dehydration
Infection
Stress: can be physical and/or emotional.
Exposure to cold

Nursing Care
Aimed at prevention and treatment of sickling episodes.
Assessment cues:-Developmental stage.
Body proportions: relationship to height and weight for age-Facial expressions.
Degree of restlessness and areas of pain, Elevated temperature, rapid weak pulse.
Weight. Loss, sunken fontanelle, poor skin turgor, dry skin, lips and mucous membranes, hydration, oxygen, pain management.

Thalassemia-Hereditary blood disorder-client cannot make sufficient adult hemoglobin abnormal size if RBC.
Several Types-most common-Beta-thalassemia has two forms.
-Thalassemia Minor- trait one parent.
-Thalassemia Major (Cooley's anemia)
Thalassemia Minor-Trait-Inherits only a gene from one parent.
Minimal symptoms-Frequently treated for iron-deficiency anemia.
S&S- pale, spleen may be enlarged, -Hgb 2-3 gm/dl lower than age related levels.
Can lead normal life- Is of genetic importance if both parents have the trait

Thalassemia Major (Cooley's anemia)-Inherit gene from both parents.
Presents with serious anemia from 6-12 months.
S&S: pale, hypoxic, poor appetite, fever, jaundice-bronze color, enlarged liver.
Treatment: multiple blood transfusions.
Prognosis: poor-death-Cardiac failure- Severe anemia.
Secondary infections.
Hemosiderosis = iron overload bronze color skin, large upper jaw.

Hemophilia- One of the oldest hereditary diseases known-deficiency in specific blood clotting factors.
Sex linked genetic patter-Males inherit from mother who is carrier.
Two Types
Hemophilia A-deficiency of Factor VIII-Most common (80%)-Recessive * know the diff between the 2.
Hemophilia B-Deficiency of Factor IX-Christmas disease*amniocentesis = option to abort.

Hemophilia-Classification:
Mild-problem after surgery or major trauma-circumcision of boys a danger of bleeds.
Moderate-bleeding episodes after trauma.
Severe-may bleed without apparent cause * 1hour to clot.
Degree of severity tends to remain constant within a given family.
S&S: not apparent in infant unless abnormal bleeding is noted, slight cut or bruise induces extensive bleeding, may show signs of shock.
Hemarthrosis cardinal sign * swelling of blood in joints.

Treatment for Hemophilia:
Replacement of deficient factor, purified or recombinant factor VII concentrates (IV- med port)
DDAVP (desmopressin) nasal spray that stops bleeding.
Parent Education- Emphasis on: signs hemorrhage.
Treatment: RICE-Rest, Ice, Compression, Elevation.
Storage and preparation of replacement factors- record keeping.
Emergency numbers and /safety equipment.
Oral hygiene, well balance meals, avoid excessive weight gain.

Regular exercise program for joint strengthening.
Avoid ASA
Observe skin for bruises or hematomas.
Keep nails short.

Idiopathic Thrombocytopenic Purpura-ITP-An acquired platelet disorder.
Most common type of purpura (purpura- a group of petechiae very circular like dark bruise.
Cause unknown-thought to be autoimmune system reaction to a viral infection.
Primary age of occurrence is between 2-4 years of age.
Manifestations of ITP
Easily bruised
Frequent nosebleeds
Recent history of rubella, rubeola or viral respiratory infection.
Platelets less than 20,000
Treatment/Nursing Care
Neurologic assessment:-Danger of Spontaneous Intracranial Bleed.
Observe for signs of bleeding-use soft toothbrush.
Limited Activity during acute stage.
Spontaneous remission occurs-6 weeks to 4 months.
Avoid drugs that interfere with platelet function.

Leukemia
Malignancy of the blood forming organs of the body that result in an uncontrolled growth of immature WBCs called blasts (stem cells)
Reticuloendothelial system is most severely affected.
Incidence is highest in 3 - 4 year olds-More common in boys.
Cause is unknown
Outside the bone marrow called extramedullary-Common sites are CNS and testicles.
Most common type of cancer in children.

Types of Leukemia -75% acute lymphoblastic leukemia (ALL)
Sudden onset & progression (2- 5 years of age) increased Blast cells.
Fever, pallor, anorexia, fatigue, anemia, hemorrhage, joint pain, splenomegaly, recurrent infection.

Acute myelogenous leukemia-(AML)-occurs more frequently in adolescents & young adults.

Spongy bleeding gums, anemia, fatigue, fever, dyspnea, moderate splenomegaly, joint & bone pain, & repeated infections.

Acute nonlymphoblastic leukemia (ANLL)-similar to AML.

Symptoms

May develop gradual or have sudden onset.

Initial phase-low grade fever, pallor, tendency to bruise, leg & joint pain, listlessness & enlarged lymph nodes, abdominal pain, constipation.

Progresses-liver & spleen enlarge.

Petechiae (Hemorrhagic spots beneath skin)

Purpura (hemorrhage into the skin) may be early subjective symptom.

S&S Blood and bone marrow test.

Treatment Chemotherapy

Given in cycles: antibiotics to prevent/control infection.

Transfusions for anemia

Sedatives: Pain relievers

Bone Marrow Transplants (BMT) and immunotherapy-Not recommended for kids with ALL in 1st remission.

Preventing infection- induction therapy reduces number of leukemic cells- harmless flora become life threatening.

Thrombocytopenia-bleeding frequent complication.

Check mouth daily for ulcers, Urinary retention, and or bleeding.

Nurse

Children's anxieties often center on their symptoms-fear of pain.

Trust is in precarious balance

Child asks if they are going to die-allow for exploration.

Private room-limit visitors

Meticulous hand washing. Observe for **S&S** of infection, dehydration, pressure sores, vomiting.

Vital Signs-check mucous membranes-Pierced body parts, skin breakdown, rectal bleeding.

Manipulate catheters gently avoid trauma to sensitive membranes.

Pain meds before pain gets out of control.

Blood must be administered with a pump. Monitor Hickman lines (Child) or mediport sites in (Teens)

Parent Education- For discharge and home care.
Avoid all Communicable diseases-Hand washing.
Nutritional Needs
High protein, calories and Fluids.
Communications with school nurse/teacher.
Soft toothbrushes, water pick, avoid commercial mouthwashes.
Alopecia from therapy.

Hodgkin's Disease-Malignancy of lymph system-Rarely seen before 5 years old.
Increased incidence adolescence and early adulthood.
More common boys than girls.
Reed-Steinberg cells present in RBC morphology X-rays, biopsy, and or body scan.
S&S-Painless lump along neck
Advanced:
Low grade fever
Anorexia
Unexplained weight loss
Night sweats
Rash/Itching
General Malaise

Treatment:
Chemotherapy and radiation
Nursing care-Relief of side effects of chemo & radiation-
Parent/Client Education.
Nursing Care of the Dying Child. Each child approaches it differently.
Inform of what you are about you do & why. Use terms they can understand.
Listen to what they say-Provide Crayons/paper for drawing.
Very therapeutic for kids-Don't forget the siblings.
Stages of dying on perceptions by age-Denial, Anger, Bargaining, Depression,
Acceptance and reaching out towards others.
*up to 9 yrs old true develop concept of death, Toddlers think they go to sleep and wake up later.

Chapter 13

Acquired Immunodeficiency Syndrome

AIDS

Human Retrovirus - ability to integrate the viral genetic make-up into the cell it infects, causing an abnormal cell that can produce more virus. Primarily attacks and cripples T lymphocytes (binds with CD4 receptor sites)
History of: chronic, recurrent, communicable diseases.
Chronic malnutrition.
Repeated contact - semen, urine, feces, vaginal secretions (sexual practices)
UN sterile instruments - tattoos, piercing.
Steroid creams as sexual lubricants.
Large number of sexual partners.

Transmission

Parenteral blood (still possible if donating before HIV antibodies can be detected), clotting factors now safe, mother-fetus.
Venereal- sexual contact (incl. oral, anal)
Possible transmission - breast milk.
None documented through casual contact - tears, saliva, CSF (cerebral spinal fluid), touching, insects.

Prevention

Public education
Detailed history with blood donation.
Blood screening test ELISA.
-Enzyme linked immunosorbent assay.
-detects Antibodies (AB) to HIV.
-Will become positive after seroconversion to HIV (6-12 weeks after exposure) up to 6 months)

Change in Lifestyle
Decreases risky behaviors
Condoms, Limit partners
No anal/oral sexual combinations.
Abstinence – the only guarantee.
Monogamy >9 years with HIV free partners.

Health Care Providers
Fear exists - treat all as potentially infected.
Ethical issue - refusal to care for AIDS patients.

Environmental
Hepatitis B lives on dry surfaces 7 - 14 days.
Risk when cleaning spills including blood, and body fluids.
1:10 bleach solution or hospital cleaning solution

Pathophysiology Agent - Human Immunodeficiency Virus.
Bloodstream - Invades cells with a CD4 molecule (leukocytes). Cells with the most CD4.
Helper T lymphocytes.
Others - Macrophages, monocytes, dendrites, microglia, retinal and Langerhans cells.

Lymphocytes
WBC differential:
Lymphocytes (increased with viral infections)
T cells, some with CD4 and some with CD8 receptors (CD4 cells fight opportunistic infections)
B cells with CD 19 receptors (mature to plasma cells that produce IgE, IgG, IgA, IgM antibodies, mutation causes multiple myeloma) - Natural Killer cells.

Process
Virus sheds its protective coating.
Exposes its core of RNA.
HIV changes RNA to DNA and becomes part of the host cell chromosomes.
As the cell reproduces, HIV is part of the permanent genetic makeup.

Clinical Stages
Exposure
Acute Retroviral Syndrome
Early Infection
Early Symptomatic Disease
AIDS

Acute Retroviral Syndrome
Seroconversion – development of HIV specific antibodies.
Presents as flu/mononucleosis symptoms – fever, lymphadenopathy, pharyngitis, HA, malaise, muscle, joint pain, nausea, diarrhea, diffuse rash, and photophobia. Occur 1 - 3 weeks (up to 6 months) after exposure, last for 1-2 weeks.
Initially, large amounts of virus found in blood.
CD4 counts decrease, then return to baseline.
HIV replication continues at a rapid, constant rate in lymph tissues (10 to the 8th power new virus each day)
Defenses
B cells initiate production of antibodies (in body fluids)
T cells initiate cellular immune response.
Antibodies decrease viral loads and T cells respond to lymph nodes, where virus is trapped.
Because T helper cells (lymphocytes) have more CD4 receptors they are affected most.

CD4 T Cells
Normal adults 800 – 1200 per microliter.
Normal life span 100 days.
HIV T cells die in 2 days.
1 billion CD4 T cells die/daily.
Bone marrow and thymus compensate by producing more T cells for years.
Early Infection
Phase may last 10 – 12 years before AIDS symptoms appear.
CD4 count > 500, remain healthy.
May have vague symptoms of HA, low grade fever, night sweats, fatigue. Maintaining normal behaviors – spreading disease.

Early Symptomatic Disease
CD4 count 200 – 499
Persistent fever, recurrent drenching night sweats, chronic diarrhea, head ache, fatigue.
Decreased immune system - localized infections, lymphadenopathy.
Infections – oral candidiasis (thrush), shingles, oral or genital herpes, vaginal candida, oral hairy.
Neuro– head ache, aseptic meningitis, cranial nerve palsy, painful myopathy and neuropathies.

AIDS – CDC Criteria
Must develop at least one of these conditions:
CD4 T cell count < 200/ microliter.
Development of opportunistic infections.
Fungal – candidiasis, Pneumocystis carinii pneumonia (cystic packs in lungs).
Viral – cytomegalovirus (CMV), herpes.
Protozoal – coccidiomycosis, cryptosporidiosis.
Bacterial – Mycobacterium TB

AIDS – CDC Criteria
Kaposi's sarcoma (rare malignant disease, tumors from connective tissue cells, travels through bloodstream - spreads through the body), Burkitt's lymphoma, immunoblastic lymphoma, primary lymphoma of brain.
Wasting syndrome (loss of more than 10percent IBM)
Dementia.

Neurological Involvement
Dementia (microglia, dendrites)
Confusion, forgetfulness, disorientation.
Loss of mental and motor function.
Speech and language dysfunction, seizures.
HIV encephalopathy, AIDS dementia.
Psychosis, stroke like condition.

Delirium

Acute confusion – disturbance in loss of consciousness, attention, thinking, perception, memory and psychomotor behavior.
Progresses rapidly (different from dementia)
Irritability, problems with sleep/wake cycle.

T Cell Function

Overall decrease and change in ratio of helper/suppressor T cell ratio (normal 2:1)

B Cell

Massive B cell activation - causes secretion of immunoglobulins.
Serum level increased, but there's no response to new antigens.
Overwhelming infections, unusual neoplasms occur.

New Saliva Test

20 minute saliva test available.
Old blood test, takes 1 week for results, have to provide counseling.
Many going undetected.

New Test – CDC Recommendations

CDC Recommendations:
Routine offering of HIV saliva tests as part of medical appointments for high risk people or those in HIV prevalent areas.
Make saliva test available to jails, homeless shelters.
Tracing partners of HIV pts, offering testing and prevention.

CDC Recommendations

Testing pregnant women, unless they refuse.
Test newborns.

Diagnostic Studies
Cellular Immune Function Tests

Absolute lymphocyte count.
T4 (helper) <300/mm (normal 800 – 1200/microliter)
Helper (T4) Suppressor (T8) ratio <1 (normal 2:1)
Electrophoresis
Increased immunoglobulins -IgG, maybe IgA, IgM.

Diagnostic Studies
Cellular Immune Function Tests
CBC decreased WBC
WBC <1500/mm
Erythrocyte sedimentation rate (ESR) >20mm/hr (normal 0 – 20)
Increases with infection or inflammation, and globulins in blood.
Skin Biopsy, Sputum C&S, lymph node biopsy.

ELISA/EIA
Done if dementia, wasting is present.
Highly sensitive enzyme immunoassay.
Screens for HIV AB (uses disrupted HIV as AG)
If blood is reactive, repeat, then confirm with Western blot test or
immunofluorescence assay (IFA)
Reactive blood x 3 = HIV antibody positive.

Western Blot Test
Electrophoresis
More expensive
Less than1percent false +

Negative Results
If high risk - repeat
May not detect in 1st 1-6 months after exposure.
May convert back to negative after AIDS has severely compromised
ability to increase AB production.
Then use clinical symptoms to diagnose.

Testing Issues
Confidentiality
Fear – loss of insurance, housing, work, relationships.
Not reported to health dept (as other STDs)
Not used to locate partners (as other STDs)
Some spread disease knowingly.
Some not competent to make decisions.
No mandatory testing

Ongoing Monitoring of Disease
CD4 counts show disease progression.
More than 500 cells - test every 3 - 6 months
Less than 500 cells - test every 2 - 3 months
200 cells – every 1 – 2 months to monitor drug treatment.

Viral Load
Quantifies amount of viral particles in serum. Also used to determine when to begin treatment, and response to drugs.
WBC - decreased, lymphopenia, thrombocytopenia (anti-platelet AB or drugs)
Anemia
Altered Liver Function Tests (LFTs) – disease and drugs.

AIDS Treatment
Combination therapy most effective in treating disease and decreasing drug resistance.
Goals:
Decreased HIV RNA to less than 50 copies/microliter (prefer below levels of detection)
Keep CD4 T cell counts to more than 200 (800 – 1200 is goal).
Delay development of HIV symptoms.

Effectiveness Measurements
Increased CD4 counts (helper T lymphocytes)
Normal > 1000
Decreased in viral load.
Risk of death increase as CD4 counts decrease, and viral loads increased (if >120,000, 71% will die in < 3 yrs)
Viral count is best predictor.
Person is still contagious even if viral level is undetectable.

Goal
To decreased viral replication for as long as possible. Virus is always reproducing.

Drug Groups

1. Nucleoside reverse transcriptase inhibitors (NRTIs)
2. Non-nucleoside reverse transcriptase inhibitor (NNRTIs)
3. Nucleotide reverse transcriptase inhibitors.
All inhibit the ability of HIV to make a DNA copy early in replication by inhibiting the activity of the enzyme reverse transcriptase.
4. Protease inhibitors (PIs) Interfere with the activity of the protease enzyme in the late stages of replication. PIs must always be used in combination, with strict adherence schedule to decrease drug resistance.
Usually 2 NRTIs and 1 PI is used together.
5. Fusion Inhibitor (Entry Inhibitor)
Work by inhibiting the binding of HIV to cells.
Resistance develops quickly if only one drug or inadequate doses are used.

Side Effects

Nausea/vomiting
Diarrhea
Tingling, pain
Sensitivity testing done to see which drugs are most effective for each patient, with fewest side effects.

Acute Retroviral Syndrome

Occurs 1-6 weeks after new seroconversion to HIV (HIV can now be detected by antibody production)
Can prevent HIV from becoming AIDS if recognized and treated aggressively (cure model)
S&S: immune response to virus.
High fever, rash, malaise, oral ulcers, lymphadenopathy.

Preventative Treatment

Treatment with drugs administered within 24 hours of exposure can prevent HIV attachment to T cells. Treatment depends on volume of the exposure and status of the source.
Need to report exposures to infection control/employee health within 24 hrs. To begin screening and immediate treatment.

Other Treatments

Interferon, interleukin 2- natural human immune proteins.
Temporary remission from Kaposi's.

Other Treatments
Pneumocystis carinii pneumonia - antibiotics
Kaposi's sarcoma - too many lesions for surgery:
Radiation temporarily effective.
Chemotherapy, alpha interferon.

Nursing Management
Teaching, prevention
Psychosocial support – loss, anger, isolation, treatment decisions.
HIV testing counseling
Drug teaching guide

Nursing Care
Nutritional support related to: wasting and diarrhea– calories,
protein, vitamins, fluids, enteral supplements, TPN
Smoking and drug use cessation
Moderate or eliminate alcohol use.
Regular exercise, adequate rest.
Stress reduction
Mental health counseling, support groups.

Dyspnea
Patients report is best indicator of distress.
Symptom of Mycobacterium TB, Pneumocystis carinii, asthma, PE,
other respiratory disorders and anemia, CHF.
Position upright, cool circulating air, O2, pursed-lip breathing,
relaxation and imagery, reassuring caregivers, music.

AIDS Dementia Complex (ADC)
From disease process, opportunistic infections, dehydration,
medication side effects.
Treat dehydration, depression, opportunistic with antiretroviral drugs

Dementia and Delirium
Nursing focuses on safety in home, reorientation, stress reduction, support for caregivers.
Reorientation may not help, may agitate them more.
Keep environment quite, soft, soothing music, keep people and surroundings consistent and familiar, family present. Windows help with diurnal cycle.

Common Complications
See disease symptoms and specific nursing care for each.
Pneumocystis carinii pneumonia.
Cryptococcal meningitis.
Cytomegalovirus retinitis.
Mycobacterium avium complex.

Chapter 14

Cancer Review

Definition

Neoplasm-Abnormal growth of tissue that is not beneficial.
Cancer-malignant neoplasm. Origin-crab-to spread out.
Carcinogenic-produces or increases chances of developing cancer-smoking.
OMA means tumor.
Sarcomas-bone, muscle & other connective tissue.
Carcinomas-epithelial tissue mouth to rectum.
Lymphomas and leukemia-blood forming organs.
Melanomas-pigment cells of the skin.

Characteristics

Benign-abnormal growth of tissue, usually harmless unless it interferes with organs normal function, encapsulated, stay in that area and do not invade surrounding tissue.
Malignant-uncontrolled rapid growth, invade surrounding tissue.
Do not look or behave like normal cells.
Nucleus is large and irregular-abnormal cell membrane-less cohesive (less sticky breaks apart easy)
Metastasize-can travel to other parts of the body where it can establish another colony.
Note: usually stays out of heart because of pressure- travels to lymph.

Etiology

Defects in the DNA of genes.
Genetics-Chemical Agents-Physical Agent-Promoters-Chronic Irritation.
Contributing Factors
Genetics (aggressive and evasive)
Genetic markers for certain types of:
Breast
Leukemia

Chemical Agents Repeated exposure to certain substance that is handled or inhaled. Petroflurocarbon .Pesticides. Smoking. Industrial wastes. Asbestos (Mesothelioma)

Physical Agent
Radiation-Viruses-Ultraviolet Rays (Melanoma is most aggressive)
Promoters
Cancer occurs at a faster rate in smokers that drink vs. smokers that do not drink.
Contributing Factors-Intrinsic factors.
Age-Sex-Race-Stress-Diet.

Prevention
Encourage patient to quit smoking.
Protective measures when using cleaning agents.
Avoid overexposure to sun.
Education the public Nutrition and no smoking.

Detection
Identification of high risk people (markers from family history)
Aggressive assessment and screening.
Screening
Breast/testicular self-examination breast exam before menses when estrogen is lower.
Stool for occult blood
Mammography
Pap-smears checks for abnormal cells and venereal diseases.
PSA prostate specific antigen (blood draw)
Diagnostic
Biopsy
Radiological Studies
X-ray
CAT

Radioactive scanning
Hot-spot
Cold
Endoscopy

Lab Tests
Alk. Phos/ PSA/Tumor markers/Pap smears-No sex 24 hours prior.

Treatment and Side Effects
Surgery
Radiation
Chemotherapy
Hormone Therapy
Immunotherapy
Gene Therapy
Surgery Types
Diagnostic - biopsy
Excising -removal
Curative-goal to cure.
Palliative comfort measures or debulk tumor.
Alopecia- hair won't grow back in targeted area from radiation.
Closer nurse is to implant greater the chance for problems.
Stay 6 ft away and 30 min a time for care.
No age under 18 or pregnant women.

Radiation/Teletherapy to pinpoint an area.

External
Nursing Care
Do not wash area with soap.
Cotton clothing-not tight.
Avoid sunlight, hot, cold.
Head and neck-use electric razors.
Side effects-3 weeks after onset subside 2 weeks after treatment.

Internal
Direct contact with tumor tissue.
Half-life
Sealed-implants
Unsealed-oral or injected.
Eliminated via secretions and excreta
Shorter half life

Nursing Care
Distance 6 ft
Time 30min
Dosimeter badge
Private Room
Patient may need to remain in bed and in certain positions.
Gloves-bedpans, linens, patient clothing-dispose according to policy.
Handle dressings with forceps.

Chemotherapy
Antineoplastic
Decrease the number of malignant cells or reduce the size of tumor.
Cytotoxic
Combining drugs
Vesicants

Side Effect
Bone Marrow Suppression
Cardiotoxicity
Neurotoxicity
Pulmonary toxicity
Hepatotoxicity
Nephrotoxicity
Ototoxicity
Other Therapies
Gene Therapy
Hormone Therapy
Immunotherapy

Common Problems and the Nursing Care
Anorexia/Mucositis-Nausea/Vomiting.
Diarrhea/Constipation-Immunosuppression.
Fatigue-Alopecia
Pain-Fear
Anorexia/Mucositis

Teach About:
Nausea/Vomiting-Reglan round clock.
Diarrhea/Constipation
Immunosuppression
Fatigue
Alopecia
Pain
Fear

Chapter 15

Vision and Hearing

Vision
Function of structures
Protection
Orbits- bone
Eyelashes- catch foreign objects.
Eyelids- protect eye
Blinking stimulates tears
Lacrimal gland- Enzymes destroy bacteria-Tears to lubricate and cleanse. Cornea assists with refraction of light.
External eyeball-sclera, choroids, retina.

Life style changes-employment, communication, interpersonal. Can't see or hear, get sensory overload easy.
Seems to be ignoring people. Increased agitation in busy surroundings.
Prevention
Basic eye care- Rest eye muscles periodically- good light for reading.
Symptoms of problems- should not see sclera-(bulging eyes) graves diseases and hyperthyroidism.
Nursing Process
Assessment- any change in vision, pain or discomfort, sudden itching, floaters, crusting, scotomata (blind spots)
History-medication taking, glaucoma, diabetes or hypertension, any reduction in vision how they adapted to it.

Tests and examinations
Visual Acuity
Ophthalmoscopy- look back of eye for blood flow.
Snellen's chart 20 ft away, normal 20/20, 20/40, 22/100 legal blind.
Tonometer- Intraocular Pressure-puffs of air how fast it bounces back to measure for glaucoma.nl 12-21mmhg.
Slit lamp- find objects-Topical dye-foreign objects or abrasions, dye and florescence light.

Nursing Diagnosis
Risk for injury related to reduced visual field.
Anxiety R/T related to loss of vision.

Stressors
Refraction- bending of light.
Myopia-lens is to close, nearsighted cant see faraway.
Hyperopia-lens is too far away- farsighted can't see close up.
Astigmatism- curvature-abnormal lens.
Presbyopia-loss of accommodation- iris muscle contract, how much light gets in goes along with pupil.
Foreign bodies- so not blink-scratches the eye-irrigate with saline or sterile water.
Prevention-Use Safety goggles.
Use of -sterile water or saline-sterile cotton swab-only swab a free floating object.
Deep imbedded-patch both eyes and go to ER- one eye follows the other is why patch both eyes.
Medication-Dyes, ointments, NSAID- decreases inflammation and pressure drops put in lower conjunctiva sac.
Put pressure on inner canthus, this decreases pressure and illuminates drops going systemic.
Ointments stay in longer- inner canthus out in the lower conjunctiva area.
Infections and Inflammation Assess-Redness, swelling of eyelid, sclera blood vessels are visualized purulent drainage.
Implement
Antibiotic eye gtt-drops. don't get a systemic effect with drops, lay head back rest side of your hand on their side of face, cheekbone or forehead for stability.

Glaucoma- too much aqueous humor.
Have: nausea, vomit, HA, tunnel vision, halo .tired eyes.
IOP-Intra ocular pressure -determined by amount of aqueous humor production.
Open angle/increased pressure, closed angle/drainage gets blocked.
S & S-mild, blurred vision, trouble adjusting to dark, narrowing vision, halos.

Diagnosis-Tonometry- puff of air to measure pressure and determine glaucoma.
Interventions
Miotic-outflow by pupil-constriction, Mydriatic is for-dilation.
Beta-adrenergic blockers.
Nurse-proper way for eye gtt/drop medication.-patient education.

Cataracts- grey pupil, poor night vision, visual glare, dim vision film on iris clouds up, common in elderly.
Chronic eye problems elderly adjust and adapt don't realize how bad the problem was.

S & S-Distorted vision, floaters photosensitivity.
Diagnosis-slit lamp.
Surgical treatment.-Removal of affected lens and implanting new lens.

Intervention-swatch for severe pain, bleeding or infection- not much pain with cataract surgery.
No coughing, sneezing, squeezing eyelids, sudden movement of head, bending at the waist, or straining for bowel movement.
These things increase intraocular pressure.
Eye shields and sun glasses, eye protection.
Eye gtt/drops-Miotic

* Good to know if your patient has had cataract surgery as pupils will not be symmetrical, will be an odd shape.

Retinal Detachment
Retinol floaters Field deficit -visual field is affected.
Flashes of light, loss of vision-sudden, cloudy vision, floaters.
Diagnosis-ophthalmoscopy
Treatment-repair hole- emergency surgery within a day or so, won't have a lot of pain or drainage.

Blindness-22/100- tunnel vision and no peripheral vision is legal blind.

Do Not Shout- Speak when entering room.

Remove hazards from environment and explain location of furniture.

Assistance with self-care- ask what they can do by themselves and what they need assistance with.

Clock method for food.

Dignity

Hearing

Ataxia-defective muscular movement.

Nerve #8 Vestibulocochlear inner ear -Labyrinth - Balance and Direction.

Prevention

No sharp instruments into canal- nothing smaller than your elbow, Q-tip just for the pinna.

Remove cerumen- enzymes to kill bacteria, use hydrogen peroxide at room temp or a little higher.

Avoid loud noise and frequency of exposure.

Avoid ototoxic drugs-when using monitor closely-do peak and trough.

Diagnosis Otoscope- visual observe.

External canal and tympanic membrane, pearly white, looking for bulging and redness.

Whisper test- behind the person.

Romberg's- equilibrium, have patient close eyes with feet together and arms out to see if balanced.

Rinne-tuning fork handle on mastoid, then by ear see where they hear better, bone conductor of sound.

If hear better mastoid means conduction loss of hearing-if hear better in ear sensory loss.

Weber-tuning fork-put handle on forehead if hear sound hearing will be normal or have a symmetrical hear loss.

Nursing Process
Assess
History-genetic when they had their hearing loss, assess medications from younger years.
Physical- outer pinna, top of ear should line up with eyes, if not sign of Down syndrome.
Inspect and palpate outer ear- a lot of lymph nodes around the ear.
Tinnitus- ASA can cause ringing,
Vertigo- dizziness and balance.

Nursing Diagnoses
Risk for injury
Knowledge deficit.
Impaired verbal communication.

Interventions
Ear gtt.-pinna up and back- straightens ear canal.
Communication- stands in front of patient.
Post-op care-assist in walking due to vertigo.
Flat in bed with head still.
Facial nerve injury-observe the eyelid dropping.
Assist until vertigo gone- use gait belt and stay with patient.
Home care-community resources for special equipment- ex light comes on when the phone rings.

Otitis Media-Inflammation of the middle ear-until 8 yrs old-because of their straight canal pathogens get in easy.
S & S-Pain-pulling on ear-red, bulging tympanic membrane.
Treatment-Antibiotics-Antihistamines.
Tympanoplasty-*put tubes in ears when all other meds don't work.

Meniere's syndrome--Increase fluid in labyrinthine spaces.
S & S-tinnitus, head ache, poor coordination, vertigo, nausea and vomiting.
Treatment-bed rest for vertigo, restrict fluids and salt.

Otosclerosis-Disease of bone in middle ear-hereditary.
S&S- begin teens-other voices muffled, own okay.
Treatment-hearing aid
Stapedectomy and insert prosthetic device- bone does not vibrate as well.
Rehabilitation and Resources.
Hearing Aids-Lip Reading.
Hearing Assistive devices- use soap and water dry thorough before turning back on and Signing- hand signs.

Chapter 16

Wellness

Wellness Is more than good health.
Defined By a person's Values, Beliefs, & Culture.
Degree of wellness varies with family community and society's beliefs. Wellness is more than absence of illness and is defined by each person. Active Process in which an individual progresses toward maximum potential Regardless of their current state.

Seven Areas of Wellness

Emotional-How the mind affects the body-Stress / Anxiety / Fear.
Mental-Coping abilities
Intellectual-Cognitive ability, Educational background.
Vocational-Job / where they live / Vehicle / Social status.
Social-Family lifestyle-Herbs / Natural / Rituals.
Spiritual-Religion / Peace within.
Physical-Developmental / Gender / Age / Race / Sex.

Behavioral Characteristics That Define Wellness

Health Promotion- Immunization, family planning, dental care, poisons control, accident prevention teaching. Health maintenance-Prevent complications (Diabetic control) Assessing growth & development.
Check-ups & Breast exams.

What is Health-Generally accepted definition from the world health organization (WHO)
State of complete physical, mental, & social well-being, not merely the absence of disease or infirmity.

What is Disease- Pathologic process with a definite set of signs & symptoms.
Diseases cause illness
May or may not be detectable.

What is Illness- Illness is a deviation from normal health.
Health status changes continually from birth to death.
Some chronic diseases or disabilities last a lifetime.
Only the person can tell you if he/she feels ill (Subjective).

Acute Illness- Rapid onset of symptoms that last a limited amount of time.

Chronic Illness- Encompasses many different physical and emotional alterations in health.
Must have one of the following:
A permanent change
Requires special client education for rehabilitation.
Requires a long period of care or comfort, 6+ months.

Causes of Illness-Invasion defenses by pathogens- Cancidas / Pseudomonas / Staph / Influenza.
Immunopathology-No passive or active immunity to the disease.

Biochemical imbalances
Exposure - Toxic substances/Hazardous environmental conditions.
Injury-Portal of entry.
Age related conditions - Arthritis
Genetic-Inherited Congenital - During 1st 6 weeks of life.

Stages of Illness
Transition stage-Onset May begin with vague symptoms & person may deny feeling ill, May self medicate.
As symptoms worsen, medical help is usually sought.
Acceptance- Sick Role Denial or illness stops, illness acknowledged, measure to get well are begun, withdrawal from normal duties.
Convalescence- Recovery-The process of returning to health begins.
Acute- Recovery may take a short period.
Chronic- Recovery may take a prolonged period.
Terminal-There may be no recovery.

Illness Prevention

Primary Prevention- Practices designed to keep health problems from developing.
Secondary Prevention- Early Detection / Screening / Diagnosis / Intervention.
Tertiary Prevention- Care for person with health problem already, prevent worsening.

Health & Illness

Current view sees people as dynamic beings.
Health states may change hour to hour.
People are located on a continuum ranging from obvious disease-Absence of disease.
Health Illness Continuum
Death-Critically ill-Illness/Poor health-mildly ill-Normal health-Good health-Highest Health.

Prevention health care Team-The individual combine's knowledge of preventive health care with behavioral changes. Nurses do initial health screening, are great teachers of preventive health habits.
Primary physicians: family doctors seen on a regular basis.

Factors Affecting Health

Genetics and human biology
Environmental influences
Personal behavior, Health care

Genetics and Human Biology

Inherited traits have an impact on an individual's state of health.
Genetic makeup may include inherited disorders or chromosomal anomalies.
Normal body functioning prevents some illnesses and makes us more susceptible to others.

Environmental Influences

Geographic location and living conditions
Natural biological irritants
Exposure to chemicals

Exposure to solar radiation
Natural disasters
Man-made crises including wars, pollution, overpopulation.

Personal Behavior

The most effect on health and wellness.
Controlled entirely by the individual.
Includes diet, exercise, personal care, sexual relationships, level of stress, tobacco drug use, alcohol use, and safety.

Health care:

Health promotion, disease prevention more effective uses for health care.
Health care should include: Physical exam Immunizations Test Dental and eye exams.

Ten Health Practices:

No tobacco or drugs.
No more than 2 ounces of alcohol per day.
Eat a low fat, low sodium, low cholesterol, high fiber diet.
Exercise regularly.
Stay lean.
Drive cars with air bags; wear seat belts; drive prudently, don't drink and drive.
Avoid excessive stress.
Minimize exposure to pollutants, and other environmental hazards.
Avoid sexually transmitted diseases.
Obtain regular medical care.

Culture and Health- Problems for nurses arise when.
Nurse's expectations are unrealistic about what the patient can or want to have done for him/her.
The type or quality of care may not be what the patient desires.
The patient's cultural beliefs are in conflict with current medical practice.
Assessment must be done without criticism.

Holistic Approach to Health-A holistic approach considers the biologic, psychological, sociologic, and spiritual needs of the person. Physical Wellness-Nursing takes a holistic approach -caring for the sick and promoting wellness.
Spiritual Wellness-Manifests itself as inner strength and peace. Spirituality is broader than religion. Spirituality involves one's relationship with self, others, the natural order, and a higher power. For many, religious practices are an expression of their spirituality. The nurse must respect the spiritual needs of their clients.

Four Areas of Self Concept:
Self Esteem: refers to how one feels about themselves as a person.
Body Image: refers to how one feels others are reacting to their appearance.
Personal Identity: refers to an individual's conscious sense of who he or she is.
Role performance: our ability to execute successfully societal expectations regarding role specific behaviors.
High-Risk Factors for Self-Concept Disturbances.
Personal identity Disturbance.
Body Image Disturbance.
Self-Esteem Disturbance.
Altered Role Performance.

Individuals do not move steadily up the hierarchy. As life situations change, needs change, and behavior is motivated by different levels of the hierarchy.

The full Meaning of Holistic care-Help clients understand how physical, intellectual, social cultural, psychological, and spiritual health is all related.

Chapter 17

Laws and Ethic Review

Important Key Words
Accountability- being responsible for ones actions.
Advocate- one who defends or pleas on behalf of another.
Customs-habits and ways of acting.
Deposition-out of court statements made by witnesses.
Ethical dilemma-no clear right or wrong answer.
Ethics- values that influence a person's behavior.
Euthanasia- letting a person die.
Informed consent doctrine-to allow a particular treatment to make an intelligent decision.
Law- how a person should act in society.
Liability- legal responsibility.
Malpractice- if one fails to meet a standard of care.
Mores-folkway- evolves from family behavior.
Negligence-situation that leads to harm to another person.
Standards of care-permitted to be preformed or prohibited from being performed.
Value clarification-self evaluation that helps a person gain insight.
Values-beliefs and worth of an object, idea, custom or attitude.
Verdict-a decision.
Abandonment of care- wrongful termination of providing patient care.
Assault-a threat to cause body harm.
Battery-intentional touching of another.
Competency-to make decisions for him/her at legal age-unless proved otherwise.
Defamation-spoken or written statements about a person that caused damage.
Harm-injury to a person.
Libel- writing about another person.
Negligence-the commission (doing) of an act or the omission (not doing) -situation to harm a person.
Slander- untrue words of another person.

Tort includes against person/ property, negligence, assault, battery, fraud.

Defendant the person liable.

Plaintiff-complaining party.

Prudent-wise.

DNR- do not resuscitate.

Key points

Laws regulate the practice of LPN/LVN and RN's.

-The patient's bill of rights and other legislation directives outline what a patient can expect from health care system.

-The LPN/LVN and RN's are legally and ethically obligated to know the scope of practice and standards of care that apply in the state where he is working.

-Every patient has the right to receive care that meets the established standards of care.

Malpractice-professional negligence is when the professional fails to meet the established standard of care.

Prevention is the best defense to a lawsuit. A competent nurse is less likely to be sued.

Ethical decisions regarding health care are influenced by a person's culture, beliefs, attitudes and values.

A code of ethics and ethical principals help guide the LPN/LVN and RN's in the practice of nursing.

Autonomy personal freedom of choice = nurse cannot make the decision for the patient.

 Beneficence- doing what is good.

Justice-what is fair.

Nonmaleficence- to do no harm.

Advance directive-is anything one wants or does not want done such as end of life care.

Legal system

Laws-prescribe how a person should act in society.

Criminal- offensive to society in general-robbery detrimental, murder assault.

Civil- person's rights.

Statutory law- developed by-fed, state, local government.

Precedent-previous ruling on an issue.

Legal process
Civil litigation-lawsuit in civil court.
Plaintiff-complaining party.
Complaint-statement by the plaintiff.
Defendant-person alleged liable.
Damages-sought by the plaintiff.
Summon-court order notifies defendant of legal action.
Answer- a detail response outline of the complaint.
Discovery-pretrial process listens to both sides.
Deposition- out of court statements by witness under oath.
Interrogatories- written questions must be answered in writing.

Verdict-decision
Appeal- request a review of the decision from a higher court to review lowers court's decision.
Deliberate- decide guilt or innocence.
Sentence- penalty.
Liability-legal responsibility.
Accountability- being responsible for ones actions.
Advocate-one who defends or pleads a cause or issue on behalf of another.

Regulation of practice
Standards of care-acts permitted to be preformed or prohibited of being preformed.
Prudent-wise
Scope of nursing practice- familiar of what he or she can do as far as practice.
Nurse practice acts-define and limit the scope of nursing practice-obtained by state board of nursing.
Interstate compact-allows multi state practice.

Legal issues
Commission- doing and act.
Omission- not doing an act.
Four elements of malpractice.
Duty exists-nurse patient establishes.

Breach of the duty-failure to perform or reasonable, prudent manner.

Harm occurs- this does not have to be physical injury.

Breach of duty was the proximal cause-of the harm-without the breach the harm would not have happened.

AHA- developed patient's bill of rights.

JCAHO- joint commission on accreditation of health care organizations- monitors health care facilities.

Omnibus budget reconciliation act- regulates any institution with federal funding.

The patient self-determination act- written policy and procedures incl. life support if incapacitated.

Informed consent—patient rights to make decisions on their health care.

Informed consent doctrine-agreement to allow a particular agreement.

Euthanasia-withholding lifesaving treatment- letting them die.

*How to avoid being sued-nurse patient relationship based on trust / respect/communication, proper documentation.

Ethics-patients values, what they believe right or wrong.

Customs-habits and ways of acting.

Culture-accepted values and beliefs of a group.

Values-personal beliefs of an object, custom or attitude.

Ethical dilemmas-do not have a clear right or wrong answer.

Ethical principles-means no one person is more important than another-autonomy-freedom of personal choice.

DNR- Do not resuscitate. Has to be written order by doctor.

Laws/ ethics

Incident report- to make data available for quality control, a tool to correct ongoing occurrences.

Never document an incident report in the charts.

Documentation: bill for services, client clinical history. All care must be documented. Neat, spellings, signed, and initialed.-, at the end of every sentence, never leave blank space, use black ink.

Medical record- legal document- and is property of the hospital.

Informed consent- must explain the common occurring risk factors: also the benefits of the procedures.

Signed consent- nurse signs to witness the patient signature only. NO patient signs if taking narcotics. Patient may have a second thought on a procedure; nurse's obligation the doc is informed to talk to them before surgery or the custodial parent signs.

Expressed consent-already given consent to the hospital for emergency care of your child while on vacation.

Implied consent-emergency treatment.

Emergency situation- life threatening procedures- 2 nurses need to sign.

Telephone consent- 2 RN's must agree, be documented and has to come in and sign the document as soon as possible.

Age of valid consent- court order, pregnant under 18.

Witness- for the patient-not a student nurse.

Against medical advice- patient can leave but must sign out leaving against medical advice.

Advanced directive document- durable power of attorney- can make a decision DNR- do not resuscitate.

Impaired nurse-substance abuse is everyone's problem.

Health care and ethics

Ethics- determine right from wrong based on knowledge not opinion.

Bioethics- general application of ethical principles: such as abortion.

Ethical principles – codes that direct and govern actions.

Autonomy- respect individual rights.

Nonmalfience-do NO harm to others

Justice- equitable distribution.

Veracity- to tell the truth.

Fidelity- do what u say you're going to do.

Value system- where we got our beliefs.

Value clarification- cannot impose your beliefs or values to a patient.

State Board of Nursing

Responsibilities
Approval of, and monitoring nursing schools; licensure.
Administers and interprets Nurse Practice Act.
Members-nurses across all levels, public member.
Appointed by governor
State Law
RN vs. LPN
Negligence-performing an act that reasonably prudent person under similar circumstance would not do.
Malpractice is negligence by professionals.

Chapter 18

Documentation Basics

Documentation and Communication in Nursing Practice.
The patient's medical record includes documentation of:
-initial assessments and reassessments.
-nursing diagnoses and /or patient's needs.
-interventions identified to meet the patient's nursing care needs.
-nursing care provided.
-patient's response to, and the outcomes of the care provided.
-abilities of the patient and/or, his significant others to manage care after discharge.
-nursing care data related to patient assessments, the care planned, nursing interventions, and patient outcomes are permanent parts of the medical record.

The purpose of Documentation supports and report that nursing action was performed and records the patient's resulting condition. Remember in a court of law if it is not documented it has not been done.

Medication Administration Documentation
When using the Medication Administration Record (MAR)
-Stay within the designated area for time and initials.
-Sign name in designated area with title and initials to the side.
-Use black ink only on the MAR.

Remember to use the **W's** when documenting on the patient chart.
-When (time)
-Why (include assessment, associated symptoms/complaints, and lab values.
-What (medication, dose, route)
-Where (site)
End your documentation with how patient tolerated the medication, including reactions and how patient was when you left.

Taking Phone Orders

If it is possible have another nurse listen to the verbal order for verification you must let the physician know someone else is on the line. Have this nurse sign the order to verify that he/she witnessed the order. Repeat the order back to the physician for clarity.
Make sure there are no blank lines in the physicians order.
Write "to" for telephone order, document the physician's name, and sign your own name. Make sure the physician signs the order within the time specified by facility policy.

Ulcer Documentation

After assessing a wound, proper documentation is necessary for medical, legal, and reimbursement reasons. Remember if it is not documented it wasn't done. If it is possible the best documentation of a wound is a photograph. Your charting should contain the following information on each wound care visit:
-Patient's name and date of visit.
-Vital signs TPR BP
-Are the dressings intact (wet, dry, loose, clean, dirty)
-Strikethrough has drainage soaked through the dressing.
-Location of wound document body area ie. Leg arm hand foot etc.
-Size of the wound length width depth in centimeters.
A sterile cotton tip applicator works well for this measurement. If there is more than one wound treat and measure each separately thus avoiding cross contamination of wounds. Compare your measurements to previous measurements to determine if wound is improving deteriorating or unchanged.
Tracking- is defined as skin overhanging a dead space.
Undermining- skin that overhangs the wound's edges.
Drainage- is there drainage on the dressing where it contacts the wound? What does it look like (serous, purulent, bloody, green, yellow, clear, thick?)
-Is the drainage part of a bio-sorbable dressing? Or is it actual drainage from the wound?
-Yellow purulent drainage could indicate staphylococcus and green could be pseudomonas. Always estimate the amount of drainage.

Odor: is there an odor from the wound which would give a great deal of information helping to identify the organism present.
-A fruity smell points toward staphylococcus and a foul fecal like would indicate a gram negative bacteria.

Necrotic tissue what percentage of the wound appears to be necrotic? Necrotic tissue should be considered as any tissue that is not beefy red and granular. Identify where the necrotic tissue is and make a small diagram.
-Infection is the wound red or streaking redness, hot and swollen? Is there soreness out of proportion to what should be present given the medical history and state of the wound? Assess infection with lab and vitals.

Classify non pressure ulcers. Wagner classification for foot ulcers. Use full or partial thickness phrasing for other types of ulcers.

Wagner Classification:
Grade 0 Pre-ulcerative lesion, healed ulcers, presence of bony deformity.
Grade-1 superficial ulcer without subcutaneous tissue involvement.
Grade 2 Penetration through the subcutaneous tissue (may expose bone, tendon, ligament, or joint capsule)
Grade 3 Osteitis, abscess, or osteomyelitis.
Grade 4 Gangrene of the forefoot.
Grade 5 Gangrene of the entire foot.

Past treatment Note the past treatments and any changes in products. This will help new health care professionals on the case. Products that may not have produced the desired results won't be accidentally duplicated.
Current treatment Document the type of irrigation, products and secondary dressings used during the dressing change.
Signature Sign the bottom of the note.
Follow up Contact the appropriate doctor, nurse, therapist or other health care professional to discuss your findings, especially if there is deterioration.

ABOUT THE AUTHOR

Carol Gibb attended nursing school as a second career after retiring from the Michigan School System. Ms Gibb had the distinction of being the oldest student nurse in her class and found it very frustrating when attending study sessions. The younger students seemed to have a language and studying style of their own that wasn't geared for the older student. Carol developed her note system and study guides which is a combination of detailed notes, key points, and keywords for all steps in nursing. This unique study guide is filled with important guidelines and information to supplement your studies, improving skills and knowledge.

 Stripping the non-essential away and leaving important facts allowed me to better memorize the systems and passing my exams. One Student Nurse To Another All in One Study Guide is a concise reference for LVN/LPN, and RN students. Finding a simple way of condensing and presenting the content facilitated the learning process that was far less confusing.

The information in this guide is intended to be a quick refresher and reference guide covering the major systems into a series of study guides. This book is the columniation of this project as a supplement to a student's current studies.

Visit us at Onestudentnursetoanother.com